I0667668

Fearless
BEAUTY
360°

A Complete Guide to
Self-Acceptance and Empowerment

KENETIA LEE

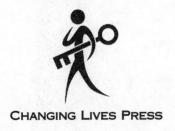

CHANGING LIVES PRESS

The information contained in this book is based upon the research and personal and professional experiences of the author. It is not intended as a substitute for consulting with your physician or other healthcare provider. Any attempt to diagnose and treat an illness should be done under the direction of a healthcare professional.

The publisher does not advocate the use of any particular healthcare protocol but believes the information in this book should be available to the public. The publisher and author are not responsible for any adverse effects or conse-quences resulting from the use of the suggestions, preparations, or procedures discussed in this book. Should the reader have any questions concerning the appropriateness of any procedures or preparation mentioned, the author and the publisher strongly suggest consulting a professional healthcare advisor.

Changing Lives Press
50 Public Square #1600
Cleveland, OH 44113
www.changinglivespress.com

Library of Congress Cataloging-in-Publication Data is available
through the Library of Congress.

ISBN: 978-0-9894529-1-5

Editor: Lisa Espinoza
Cover and interior design: Gary A. Rosenberg • www.thebookcouple.com

Printed in the United States of America

10   9   8   7   6   5   4   3   2   1

Contents

INTRODUCTION

What Makes a Woman Feel Beautiful?

It was a cool, brisk March morning in Upstate New York. Revlon cosmetics had selected eight of us makeup artists to go on a 25-city tour across America to promote their new mascara, Fabulash. I remember it like it was yesterday—the excitement and anticipation. We set up all of our makeup stations 30 minutes before the mall even opened and then huddled in a group to talk about what this tour might mean for our careers. As a freelance makeup artist, I was almost certain this would be a game changer for me. But I was even more excited about the opportunity to meet so many different women from around the country. It was my love for people that had been the driving force behind my desire to be a makeup artist in the first place.

I distinctly remember the first woman who sat in my makeup chair. She had long, brown hair, hazel eyes and beautifully sculpted cheekbones. "My name is Kenetia, and today I can show you how to play up your favorite feature. What is one of your favorite facial features?"

"Well, nothing really."

"I find that hard to believe. What about your eyes? You have beautiful hazel eyes. Let's start there." She was pleased with the outcome.

She smiled as she looked in the mirror, took her free goodies and went on about her day.

About 15 minutes later, another woman sat down in my chair. Her skin was as smooth as porcelain, and her smile could light up a 30-foot well. She seemed genuinely delighted, so I asked her a slightly different question. "How would you like me to accentuate your best feature?" She replied, "I really hate my skin. Can you please show me which foundation would work the best to make my skin more even?"

I tried to hide my confusion—her request shocked me. Her beautiful skin was the first thing that I had noticed about her. As I started to look for foundation to match her skin tone, I asked, "What are you wearing on your face right now?" She replied, "Nothing." Completely bewildered, I found her a foundation color that was an exact match to her skin tone, and, although the sheer application was not a significant change from before, she appeared to be satisfied.

By about two hours into my first day, I had heard: "Will you make my nose appear smaller? It's hideous!" "Can you make my eyes look bigger? They are so small and make me look sad." "I don't know what you are going to do with this face. I can't stand to look at it!" "Do you have a magic wand in those makeup brushes? Cuz you're going to need it."

Nine out of ten women who sat in my chair had nothing good to say about their looks. For three months, eight hours a day, I engaged hundreds of different types of women with similar requests. Their negative commentary was jarring, but admittedly, it was very similar to how I always complained about my own appearance. I didn't get it. Not one of the women that I encountered was an eyesore. All were, in fact, quite pleasing to the eye. So why was their commentary about themselves so harsh and demeaning? What would it take for these women to feel beautiful?

> Nine out of ten women who sat in my chair had nothing good to say about their looks.

Challenging Women to Embrace Their Beauty

From that point forward, I committed my life to understanding beauty —true beauty that isn't dependent on makeup techniques or youth or perfection. That's what Fearless Beauty is about. It is a movement that challenges women to embrace their uniqueness. Fearless Beauty is a way of thinking and being that leads to a shift in your relationship with your appearance. By putting into practice the ideas and exercises in *Fearless Beauty 360°*, you will learn to recognize, cultivate and celebrate the beauty that you already possess.

> *By putting into practice the ideas and exercises in* Fearless Beauty 360°, *you will learn to recognize, cultivate and celebrate the beauty that you already possess.*

I chose the word "fearless" because it is both a powerful and an empowering term. It suggests the strength, centeredness and capability to achieve anything. You possess—and you *deserve* —this quality. We will uncover it and nurture it throughout this book.

The words "fearless" and "beauty" may seem like they don't quite fit together. When it comes to your appearance, you may be more "fearful" than "fearless." Your happiness or lack of satisfaction with your appearance manifests itself in many aspects of your life: your mood, your relationships, your everyday choices and your potential. Many of the women at my Revlon station who expressed displeasure about their appearance showed it in how they carried themselves and how confidently they communicated. This often changed after I finished applying their makeup and discussing how attractive they actually were. Over time, I would learn that improving a person's self-image is the most direct way to help them feel better about their appearance.

What This Book Does (and Does Not) Offer

Fearless Beauty 360° is designed so that you experience personal reward as you move through the book and through each chapter of your journey. As you will find, the rewards grow in scope and impact along the way. *Fearless Beauty 360°* will:

- Reveal the cost of chasing physical beauty, so you can determine whether your current efforts are worth your investments of time, money and energy. (Chapter 1)

- Enable you to uncover your self-sabotaging, internal dialogue that keeps you searching for that one elusive *thing* that will fix your perceived imperfections. (Chapter 2)

- Expose how the past has shaped your self-image. (Chapter 3)

- Assist you in disengaging from strong negative emotions that keep you bound to your past. (Chapter 4)

- Supply you with the tools to help you let go of anything that does not represent your truest expression. (Chapters 4, 5 and 6)

- Give you the courage to listen to your intuitive voice and accept yourself. (Chapters 6 and 7)

- Show you how to create your beauty on your own terms in a way that is balanced and sustainable. (Chapter 8)

- Demonstrate how adding simple practices to your normal schedule will keep the Fearless Beauty in you alive and well. (Chapter 9)

- Provide you with a daily beauty ritual that will strengthen your intuitive voice and build confidence. (Chapter 10)

Fearless Beauty 360° will not give you the recipe for the perfect body, teeth, skin, shape or hair. It will not tell you what makeup or clothing brings out your best features, and it will not give you advice about the best exercise program for staying fit throughout your life. While all of these things can play an important role in helping you feel confident about your appearance, they are simply outcomes. When your internal dialogue is one of self-love, you will naturally incorporate those items into your life that are most nurturing.

This book is also about a woman's journey to self-acceptance—of stepping out from underneath limiting beliefs and into greatness. Everything you will read here comes from my personal struggles and from my interactions with hundreds of women from around the world. These women taught me that looking good takes a lot of effort, but beauty is simply a state of being. The goal of this book is to make feeling beautiful accessible without dependence on external factors.

> *. . . everything you need in order to be the highest expression of yourself comes from within you.*

You Are an Expert in You

Countless studies, books and documentaries offer an airtight case for how the world, media and advertisements cause women to have low self-esteem and to feel objectified. Certainly, knowing how society plays a role in diminishing your self-image is valuable information. However, I have found that blaming others makes it difficult to assume responsibility for the way I feel about myself. Blaming also impedes our ability to focus on the necessary changes that can move us toward empowerment.

In this book, I will use a process grounded firmly in the belief that everything you need in order to be the highest expression of yourself comes from within you. Much of what you will discover as you proceed through this book will be rooted in your growing awareness of self.

Over the years, I have participated in a number of transformational self-improvement courses. Not all of these courses were pleasant at the time, but each one has positively affected my life in a significant way. I have also read great books, taken amazing classes and enjoyed wonderful retreats that immediately shifted my self-perspective. Each time, it seemed that within weeks, I was back to my usual, dismal self-image. I believed that a book, course or retreat would fix my current situation, similar to how many women with whom I worked believed that new cosmetics, clothes or plastic surgery would improve the low self-esteem that they believed stemmed from dissatisfaction with their appearance. Through my exploration to know myself better, I have learned that the *journey never ends.* We are always growing and learning and changing to be the best, truest expressions of ourselves.

Until my visit to a meditation center, it did not occur to me that I needed to *incorporate* what I had been learning into my daily life. The "transformational high," as I call it, would always wear off because I had not yet learned to sustain my new discoveries through a daily practice that would expand on what I had learned.

Because of this realization, I begin each exercise in this book with a short meditation to help ground you. This will open you to the concept of "going within" and allow you to realize your own answers.

The Way of a Fearless Beauty

A Fearless Beauty is constantly moving in the direction of her desires, which means first knowing what she wants and then taking actions consistent with those wants. You will learn my daily beauty ritual that enables me to appreciate my unique talents, gifts and beauty and allows me to overcome the pressure to be, act or look like someone other than me. Since accepting the way of a Fearless Beauty, countless people have stopped me and made comments like, "Whatever it is you have, you need to bottle it up and sell it! Everyone is looking for a little bit of whatever *that* is!"

I believe that these people are referring to my presence and unwavering confidence. I wouldn't have either of these qualities if I did not maintain the daily beauty ritual I refer to as Fearless Beauty. Fearless Beauty is not *THE* answer. It is simply one way for you to find *YOUR* answers and to experience a profound sense of well-being that frees you to fully embrace and express your unique embodiment of beauty.

Welcome to the journey!

CHAPTER 1

Looking Good—
What Really Stands Between
You and What You Desire

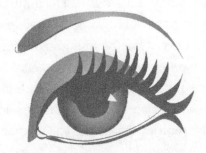

Looking good takes a lot of effort,
but beauty is simply a state of being.
—Kenetia Lee

My Experience Fueled My Mission

When I was a little girl, my mother wanted to earn some extra money for an overseas trip to visit her sister. After looking into a few possibilities, she decided to invest $100 to become a Mary Kay beauty consultant. My mother was ecstatic as she explained her new enterprise to my father, and I couldn't help but be excited for her. This was the moment when my fascination with beauty began. I knew then that I would be the best nine-year-old assistant beauty consultant ever.

It was a big day for us when our new consultant's case arrived. I watched, eyes as wide as saucers, as my mother opened up the first box of promotional products. I immediately began helping her fill the pink promotional makeup cases that came with her order. By the time she had opened all of her boxes, we had a huge pile of sample makeup, lipsticks, cleansers and moisturizers. It was like being in a department store, but right there in our living room. What was even better, as far as I knew, it was all free!

This was my introduction to makeup. I didn't have a clue about what all this stuff was supposed to do, but it didn't matter. My mom was excited about it, and that was enough for me. Aspiring to be the perfect assistant, I began to practice setting up the demonstration trays. Within a few days, we did our first beauty consultation, and I watched in amazement as four women I had never met listened intently and followed every one of my mother's beauty instructions. After the demonstration ended, they ordered various lipsticks and eye shadows and remained loyal customers for years.

It seemed like each group we worked with enjoyed themselves immensely while my mother shared her valuable beauty advice. They bragged about how wonderful her products made their skin feel, and I had a blast playing along as if I were one of the women in my mother's group. My favorite part was applying those miniature, M&M-shaped lip colors to my small, pursed lips with the accompanying disposable lip brush.

Although I enjoyed playing with the various moisturizers and makeup samples, I did not understand what inspired these women to spend so much money on beauty products. I wanted to know what made them so happy, so quickly. I knew that in order to figure it out, I would need to pay more attention at future consultations. After weeks of watching my mother work with various customers, I came to learn that my mom was not just selling skin-care advice or new cosmetics. She was selling the hope of feeling more youthful and attractive.

Clients would talk to my mother about what they had lost in recent relationships, how tired they felt, how little time they had to themselves, and how they were never able to do the little things for themselves that made them feel good. Some of their stories would even bring me to tears.

My mother excelled at her job and offered fabulous makeup advice.

But more importantly, she had a gift of gab that often left these women not only feeling good about their appearance, but also feeling empowered to change their current circumstances. When my mom finished a demonstration, most of the women she spoke to displayed an obvious shift in how they felt about their beauty. Their shoulders relaxed; their backs straightened. They were smiling. Many even spoke with more confidence and acceptance of their looks than they had at the beginning of the demonstration.

This was the beginning of my journey to discover the secret of beauty—real beauty. I wanted to empower women and make them feel as happy as my mother did. To that end, right out of college, I worked as an aerobics instructor at a women-only gym. Then, I moved to California and took a few courses to pursue a career in the entertainment industry as a makeup artist. After completing my courses, I worked as a makeup artist for Smashbox Cosmetics at the Mercedes-Benz Fashion Week in Los Angeles. Soon thereafter, I accepted a management position at L'Oreal Paris's first retail store.

I have dedicated my entire career to learning all I can about physical beauty. But it wasn't until I faced major breakdowns in my relationships, my health and my career that I began to seek out a deeper understanding of beauty. These challenges left me feeling downright hopeless, desperate and truly ugly. I was my harshest critic, seeking out every product on the market that might help me feel good about the person I saw in the mirror.

I collected thousands of lotions, pills, creams, ointments, gels and scrubs in an attempt to make my hair and skin more luscious, thicker, stronger, brighter and softer. Had I taken an inventory of my assortment of beauty enhancers, I could have opened my very own beauty department! I had a product for everything you could imagine, each promising to make me look just a little bit better. I bought them with the hopes that I would feel whole.

I was a self-proclaimed "improvement junkie," spending hours and hours, month in and month out, rummaging through *Vogue*, *Elle* and

InStyle magazines looking for some sort of answer to my latest beauty dilemma. I needed some way to mask the discontentment I felt about my appearance and about my life as a whole. I characterized my appearance in much the same way that my Revlon clients catalogued their flaws. Like many of my mother's Mary Kay customers, I was on a continual search for the next product or technique that would revolutionize how I saw myself. But despite all my best efforts, I did not feel any more attractive or empowered than when I began.

Shouldn't We Feel *More* Beautiful?

With so many beauty enhancements at our disposal, including plastic surgery, and significant social and political advances made by women over the past century, how is it possible that women are not feeling more empowered concerning their self-image? Naomi Wolf, political activist and author, notes in *The Beauty Myth* that "women have more money, power, scope and legal recognition than ever before. . ." This is no empty statement. Less than a century ago, women did not even have the right to vote. Now, women are poised to become the most powerful demographic in the United States economy.

Citing a report released by the United States Census Bureau in early 2012, Richard Perez-Pena reveals that women are about to surpass men in attaining undergraduate and graduate degrees.[1] Also, in an article titled "The top 30 stats you need to know when marketing to women," Ekaterina Walter provides ample evidence that women are economically more powerful than ever before. She notes that women currently control 60 percent of all private wealth in the United States and that analysts expect the average American woman to earn more than the average American male by the year 2028.[2]

Women have clearly made great advancements over the past century. Yet we still struggle with our image. Much like me years ago, the average woman invests a small fortune on her looks each year. In 2007, surgical and nonsurgical cosmetic procedures rose 457 percent from the previous 10 years combined.[3] In 2010, women spent a total of $59 billion on beauty products in the United States.[4] Even at the young age of nine, I witnessed this trend with my mother's customers—spend, spend, spend in order to be beautiful.

In spite of all of these appearance upgrades, a recent study by the Dove Foundation revealed that only 2 percent of women use the word "beautiful" to describe their appearance.[5] Considering the volume of beauty enhancements American women indulge in, this is a truly bleak statistic. Wolf surmises, in terms of "how women feel about themselves *physically,* they may actually be worse off than their unliberated grandmothers!"[6]

If only 2 percent of women would describe themselves as beautiful, what is going on with the other 98 percent?

As I gained more experience as a makeup artist and grew more comfortable in my role as a beauty expert, I became more of a makeupologist—a cross between a makeup artist and a psychologist. As my mother did with her customers, I asked more intimate questions about why each woman expressed such harsh commentary about her looks. I found that they tied most of their negative perceptions to deeper internal issues rather than to their latest beauty woes.

Who or What Shall We Blame?

Are the media, fashion and corporate conglomerates to blame for our declining appreciation of unique beauty and the self-deprecating, consumer-driven narcissism that result?

It is true that the media and the beauty industry exploit the public's desires and fantasies with their portrayal of beauty in advertising and entertainment. An advertiser's job is to convince women that their product or service will bring happiness, adoration and even love in the guise of pearly white teeth, bigger breasts or less wrinkles. These skillfully crafted messages keep women hoping for that which they feel is ultimately missing from their lives.

The reality is, advertisements do not create these thoughts of incompleteness. Unhappy thoughts that define what is missing from a woman's life take root in her psyche well before advertising messages arrive. Thus, women can do little to change the effectiveness of these insidious marketing practices if they do not first address their personal fears concerning beauty. In her book *Reality Bites Back,* Jennifer Pozner says, "The advertising industry is a $200 billion a year industry specifically focused on crafting and delivering messages for us to consume. However crafty the media is, we are not at a point where we will completely suspend our rational thought process or belief system."[7] *I am sure they are working on it though!*

If the under-appreciation of one's own unique beauty is an issue of blame, plenty of other scapegoats exist. Women could definitely blame men for using women's bodies and images as means for sexual pleasure. The objectification of women in contemporary society is undeniable. Additionally, parents could account for some, if not most, of the anxiety many women develop in relation to their self-image. Women could also blame cruel kids who made them feel like outcasts during their teenage years.

The truth is, as long as women are playing the "blame game," they will not be in a position to face their fears and learn to embrace their God-given beauty, talents and abilities. In addition to suspending blame, it is also imperative that women find sustainable habits and behaviors to promote a healthy self-image. We will talk about how these habits come together to form our beauty ritual as we advance through the book.

Temporary Fulfillment

My experience tells me that a woman's pursuit of physical perfection brings only temporary fulfillment. No matter how much we do to improve our physical appearance, unless we address our deeper desires for acceptance, appreciation and self-worth, we will continue chasing the delusion that something we put on or do to our faces or bodies will ultimately fulfill us and make us feel as beautiful as we long to feel. It's no wonder that at the end of the pursuit, women often feel more frustrated and hopeless because their physical enhancements and improvements do not change their self-perception to the core. And the cycle of negative self-image continues.

In order to transform how we perceive and value our appearance, women need to develop the skills necessary to identify the triggers that fuel our feelings of unworthiness. These triggers could be as trivial as television commercials for stronger, thicker nails or devices that give you flatter abs in six days. Triggers may also be more personal, such as tragic or devastating news. Your husband telling you that he is having an affair, learning that you will not get the job for which you interviewed six times or realizing that you are no longer able to fit into your favorite pair of jeans could all serve as personal triggers.

These triggers—trivial or tragic—are simply reminders of lingering pain from your past that needs to heal. You can cover up that pain by spending money on a new pair of shoes or dying your hair. You can go to the makeup counter, where a lovely representative will affirm how beautiful you are and assure you that you *absolutely* need their new face cream to make you look flawless.

Some consumerist attempts to solve beauty issues are harmless, except to the pocketbook, and yield only temporary results. Other related tactics, however, can be extremely harmful to your health and result in long-term negative consequences. It might not be surprising to learn that 67 percent of women between the ages of 25 and 45 in the United States (excluding those with actual eating disorders) are trying to lose weight. What *is* alarming, however, is that 53 percent of these dieters are already at a healthy weight.[8] Additionally, nearly 10 million women in the United States suffer from an eating disorder, such as anorexia or bulimia, and show signs of having low self-esteem.[9] Many women cite that a desire to be healthier is their main reason for wanting to lose weight. However, according to a recent study undertaken by the University of North Carolina at Chapel Hill and *Self* magazine, 13 percent of women smoke to lose weight.[10] Despite the fact that smoking is directly responsible for 90 percent of all lung cancer deaths in the United States each year,[11] many women ignore obvious dangers in their pursuit of what they perceive as beauty. By pursuing means that at the least bring only temporary satisfaction and at the most bring negative health consequences, women often undermine themselves in the pursuit of beauty.

For decades, women have been at the source of great change and equality in the United States. I believe that we will make even greater strides at an even faster rate as we become empowered by our unique expression of self. We can, will, and must force positive changes in how the media depicts women, how companies advertise to women and how local, state and national government legislation affects the well-being of women in this country. Nevertheless, this is not where the process begins. *It starts with you.*

As we move through this book, I will help you distinguish those triggers that may set you off, find the deeper beliefs that you have about yourself and show you how to use forgiveness to move beyond the pain from your past. Attempts to find your beauty through means of temporary fulfillment will become less of a task and more enjoyable as well. The alternative is to keep looking outside of yourself, fixing what is not actually broken and constantly pointing the finger at outside entities that have no power to bring about the change you are seeking within yourself. This search for beauty through means of temporary fulfillment only perpetuates the awful fear that you are not good enough just as you are. Please, hear me now—this is simply not true. You are good enough right now, this moment.

Three Beauty Blocks

I remember how much better my mother's Mary Kay customers felt after having conversations that delved deeper than what cosmetics they should purchase. Once I became a professional makeup artist, I began to realize how skilled women were at avoiding deeper issues of dissatisfaction with relationships, health and well-being by misdirecting their attention to their physical appearance—an issue that my makeup brushes alone did not have the capacity to fix. Intellectual awareness aside, these women were looking to transform the way they felt by fixing their façade.

Over the years, I have identified three common blocks that keep women from acknowledging their beauty:

Block #1: Conflict and unresolved issues from past relationships. These situations often erode self-esteem, causing women to feel unattractive or even ugly. Such emotional unrest leads to a negative perception of one's appearance.

Block #2: Unrealistic ideals based on comparisons. These women decide how they should or should not look based on where they are in their lives. They look to their past, next-door neighbors, airbrushed models, honed and pampered actors and anybody they can use to make themselves feel unworthy.

Block #3: Neglect of holistic self-care. They spend an inordinate amount of time, energy and money on their physical appearance but overlook the necessity to nurture and care for their emotional and spiritual well-being. This neglect leaves women feeling depleted, out of balance and less than attractive.

By addressing these three blocks head-on, it is indeed possible to stop this beauty war that women wage with themselves. If this is accomplished, the incessant desire for beauty enhancements (which often carry great risks) could become a thing of the past, and women would become much more likely to acknowledge themselves as naturally beautiful and capable of achieving whatever they desire regardless of what they look like.

Facing Your Biggest Fear

As Deepak Chopra famously teaches in *The Seven Spiritual Laws of Success,* "Our essential nature is one of pure potentiality."[12] This includes your ability to choose how you interpret and use your life experiences and how you perceive your physical appearance. There is really no one to blame for the way you feel about yourself—*not even you.* When you are capable of facing the events in your past, as well as the people who planted any fearful notions in your head that you are not pretty or good enough, you will be able to mold your pure potential.

> *There is really no one to blame for the way you feel about yourself—not even you.*

Blame, as I have come to learn, is just another convenient way to avoid taking responsibility for your feelings. You must own your feelings before you can change them. Being stuck in this place of blame is your greatest indicator that you are seeking to experience something more or different than is currently in your life. It's a wake-up call, if you will, and an opportunity to let go and expand.

Let go of what, you ask?

• Thoughts, beliefs or feelings that you don't measure up or are inadequate in any way

• Shame, blame or guilt that you feel about your body and limitations

• Past stories, people, events, activities or circumstances that make you feel insecure and self-conscious

• Character traits, behavior patterns, ideals or activities that keep you stuck in a holding pattern, continuously chasing an idealized body of perfection, instead of allowing you to feel good about yourself

Until you are able to overcome blame and face the fears of your past, you will continue to chase an artificial concept of beauty instead of pursuing your life's ambitions. The voice in your head will haunt you

16

with questions that diminish your worth, such as, "Who am I to be brilliant, stunning, gifted or beautiful?"

As Marianne Williamson said, "Who are you *not* to be? You are a child of God. Your playing small does not serve the world. There is nothing enlightened about shrinking so that other people don't feel insecure around you. We are all meant to shine, as children do. We were born to make manifest the glory of God that is within us. It's not just in some of us; it's in everyone. And as we let our own light shine, we unconsciously give other people permission to do the same. As we are liberated from our own fear, our presence automatically liberates others."[13]

I first read Williamson's full quote when I was 15. At that time, I did not comprehend exactly what she was saying, but I knew in my heart that there were truths within this statement that I wanted to know as *my* truth.

How do you face your fears about your own light and become more of who you are instead of relying on more of the same unsuccessful tactics?

You Have the Power

Are you in a cycle of fear that compels you to look or be something other than who you are? Restore your power by taking responsibility for the feelings and behaviors you have developed that do not empower you. Once you have done this, align yourself with what feels authentic rather than being a victim of your circumstances.

When you assume responsibility for how you respond to your situation, you have the kind of power that no one can take away, regardless of what life throws at you. Those silly commercials that try to convince you that you are incomplete without their product will also have no effect on you.

According to Suzanne Reisman, "If women collectively decided that we were fine with our faces without makeup enhancing them, it would certainly cost the American economy an enormous amount of money and thousands of jobs would be lost."[14] In other words, if we as women loved ourselves as we are, we would have a direct negative effect on the profits of the beauty and cosmetic industries. Are you shocked to hear this from someone who is a career makeup artist? Believe me, I'm not suggesting that you should completely reject caring for your physical bodies or suspend your use of all cosmetic and beauty products. I know very well that lotions and potions are truly enjoyable and, in some ways, help connect you with your feminine energy.

How you feel about your beauty is up to you.

However, it is important to understand that your *power* to *feel beautiful* is not *dependent* on the products marketed by beauty, fashion and other corporate conglomerates.

Though advertisers bombard you with the message that their products will fix you, you are not broken. How you feel about your beauty is up to you. If lotions, potions, clothes or makeup are your primary resource for emotional and spiritual fulfillment, you are living in a disconnected state from your true self.

Instead of looking at others for quick beauty solutions, begin your search for beauty by going within and asking yourself questions about what beauty really means to you. When I stopped relying on the outside world to dictate my definition of beauty and started defining beauty for myself, I experienced greater, farther-reaching rewards than any ultra-whitening toothpaste or push-up bra could have ever offered.

You Are the Real Influencer

Taking back my power has not stopped the media or society from objectifying the female body, but it has given me peace of mind and a desire to share what I have learned. I now have a passion to carry my message to younger women so that they can begin to live fulfilled lives without some of the struggles that you and I have experienced with regard to self-acceptance.

When you start to take back your power, an immediate by-product is that you make a powerful difference in the lives of younger, impressionable girls. Young women, such as your daughters, sisters, cousins and next-door neighbors, pay attention to how you value yourself and will tend to mimic what they learn from you. Your behavior and attitude about your appearance directly impacts how these women see themselves. In fact, you influence their choices even more than the media. Your ability to accept yourself and your beauty will ultimately affect them in a positive way.

By setting a positive example for young women, you enable them to have a healthier relationship with their image, break through glass ceilings, eradicate discrimination and conquer uncharted territory. We have paved the way for young girls to make their mark in the world. Now we have to help them embrace and appreciate the women they see in the mirror each day.

Those closest to you are your greatest role models for how you should love and respect yourself. Others are watching how you treat yourself, even if you do not realize it. By making a few shifts in how you relate to your beauty, it is possible to change how other women relate to themselves.

Instead of looking at others for quick beauty solutions, begin your search for beauty by going within and asking yourself questions about what beauty really means to you.

For instance, if you are critical of what you wear or how your hair looks every morning, it will eventually lead those younger women who witness this self-dialogue to act in similar ways. Instead of saying, "These pants make me look fat," say, "I think the other pair might complement me better." The delivery makes all the difference.

Let your female protégé know that we all have setbacks and shortcomings and that these are all natural occurrences to be worked through, not to be derailed by. Debunk stereotypical myths about her worth when you are at the grocery checkout line and see magazine covers displaying half-naked pictures of airbrushed models. Be open to talking with young women about what they see and hear on a daily basis. Help them engage in honest dialogue about what beauty actually means to them.

Preparing for Your First Beauty Exercise

Throughout the book, you will encounter a number of exercises meant to guide you through the process of becoming a Fearless Beauty. Each exercise begins with a short period of quiet time designed to help you focus on the topic at hand. I refer to this as meditation. If meditation is completely new to you, it is important to understand that what you will be doing is not related to any religion. If you choose to do so, you can certainly use meditation to enhance your religious or spiritual practices; however, the practice of meditation, as employed in this book, is simply a matter of quieting your mind.

Meditating is a powerful way to focus your thoughts on your present circumstances. It will help you release any thoughts and feelings that may distract you from your beauty exercise. Consider this quiet time a temporary reprieve from your daily wear and tear. Meditation has proven to be the most effective way to hear your intuitive voice. When done on a consistent basis, answers to untold beauty secrets arise. Choices that help you achieve your goals will become clearer.

Before I learned to meditate, the longest amount of time I was ever quiet was the brief period in bed before I fell asleep. My mind was always racing, thinking, wondering, figuring things out and planning what I wanted to do next.

During my first meditation, I felt quite silly. I sat in a circle with a group of people doing absolutely nothing. My mind raced about 1,000 miles a minute. Every few minutes, I would peek at the other people in the circle and wonder if they were looking at me too!

After a few days of meditation, the chatter in my mind slowed down, and I started to enjoy myself. It felt good to let go of the world for a few minutes a day. By the time I left the meditation class, I was determined to make meditation a part of my daily life.

The effects of meditation on your body, mind and spirit are so expansive that there are whole sections in bookstores dedicated to the subject of meditation. Despite all of the information that I have read about meditation, my experience has been the greatest teacher. Meditation has given me the insight to accept my imperfect perfections. It has also enabled me to forgive others and myself. Best of all, meditation has allowed me to love the little girl within me and the woman she continues to become.

Meditation will not make your nose smaller or your lips poutier—at least I don't *think* it will! But it will have a tremendous impact on the way you feel about yourself. Regular meditation leads to calmness, inner peace and lower stress levels.

How to Meditate

Here are a few suggestions to help you enjoy quiet meditation time:

- **Find a quiet area where there will be no disturbances.** This could be a corner of a room or, for some, a closet, garage, basement or garden.

- **Wear comfortable, loose clothing.** If you are away from your normal place of meditation and cannot change clothes, be sure that none of your clothing is pinching or pulling on you in a distracting way.

- **Use a timer.** This could be a cell phone, watch or alarm clock. I typically meditate for 30 minutes, but that may seem like an eternity for someone who is just learning to meditate. Set your timer for five minutes your first time. As your comfort level increases, increase your meditation time by five minutes.

- **Breathe.** Remember to breathe in through your nose and out through your mouth. If it helps to quiet your mind, focus on your breath.

- **Sit in a comfortable position.** Do not let physical limitations get in your way while meditating. If possible, sit in a comfortable, cross-legged position with your hands on your knees and your back straight. If this does not work, sit in a comfortable chair with your back upright, or lie on your back on a flat surface.

Warning: If you get too comfortable, you may fall asleep. If you find yourself falling asleep the first few times you meditate, it could be a sign that your body is tired and needs more rest than it is getting. Do not let this stop you from continuing the practice of meditation. Have compassion for yourself, and allow the practice to unfold on its own.

The more clearly you are able to communicate what beauty is to you and why you want to feel beautiful, the closer you are to realizing your desire to feel authentically beautiful.

Let's start developing our beauty ritual by doing the exercise on page 23. Your answers to these questions will guide you through the course of this book. The more clearly you are able to communicate what beauty is to you and why you want to feel beautiful, the closer you are to realizing your desire to feel authentically beautiful.

There are no wrong answers, so please feel free to answer from your heart. I have asked hundreds of people these three questions, and I have never gotten the same answers. This leads me to believe that beauty is whatever YOU say it is. Remember, you have the power. Use it.

Exercise: Ask Yourself about Beauty

- **Location:** A quiet place where you will not be disturbed

- **Materials:** A pencil or pen and a timer

- **Set your timer for:** 10–15 minutes of uninterrupted time

- **Preparation:** Take five minutes to go within and quiet your mind.

- **Instructions:** Once you have completed your preparation meditation, please answer the following questions. Do your best not to sensor yourself. Whatever comes to mind, write it down. If you want to make a list instead of writing your answers in paragraph form, do that. Do not stop writing until the alarm goes off on your timer.

  ○ What is beauty?

  ○ Why is feeling beautiful important to you?

  ○ What obstacle stands in the way of your feeling beautiful now?

CHAPTER 2

Damaging Effects of Your Internal Diva's Dialogue

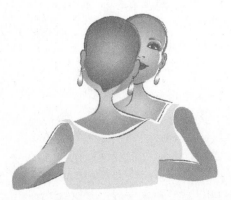

Yes, there are times when something is legitimately not our fault. Blaming others, however, keeps us in a stuck state and is ultimately rough on our own self-esteem.

—Eric Allenbaugh

Herstory: How Do You Perceive Your Physical Beauty?

The consumer behaviors discussed in Chapter 1 prove how much importance women place on looking good—and feeling good—about the way they look. What is preventing women from actually *experiencing* satisfaction from all of their efforts?

A Dove Foundation study concluded that how women feel about their beauty is directly related to how they feel about their life relationships.[1] Therefore, a woman's perception of her appearance is positive or negative based on how she feels about her relationships, past and present. We will dismantle this first beauty block by analyzing those relationships that may have significantly influenced your perception of yourself.

I have found that almost every woman with whom I have inter-acted—myself included—who has a negative self-perception is plagued by what I call a "Herstory." Your Herstory is a chronicle of past events that has played a significant role in shaping your self-image. It is the story you tell yourself about who you are and what your capabilities are. You can view your experiences as positive or negative, dishearten-ing or uplifting, remarkably dramatic or irritably annoying. Regardless of how you view these events, they have drastically affected your self-perception. Some common questions that often reveal elements of your Herstory are:

- Did your friends or classmates compare you unfavorably to your sis-ter when you were young?

- Did your dad fail to acknowledge you for things you felt you did well or when you thought you looked your best?

- Was your family or community obsessed with appearances, or did they view such superficial concerns with disdain?

- Did your mom talk negatively about her appearance or body weight in front of you?

- Were you labeled a tomboy, a princess, a geek, or an average girl?

These questions may highlight moments that made you question whether or not you were acceptable.

On the other hand, if you grew up as the center of attention, show-ered with compliments because of your physical appearance, you may have developed an intense infatuation with beauty or even an extreme case of vanity. These experiences can drive a woman away from true beauty and closer to becoming the Evil Queen, demanding praise as in the story Snow White.

Every Herstory leaves impressions that nestle in your mind and distort your self-image.

Whatever the circumstances of your past, the meaning and implications of your experiences are very real. You may have turned your perceptions about what happened to you in the past into an elaborate story to justify or defend against its painful effects.

This becomes your Herstory, and it is not necessarily isolated in the past. Every Herstory leaves impressions that nestle in your mind and distort your self-image. A person's self-image is a mental picture, generally resistant to change, which depicts details often available to others' objective investigation (e.g., height, weight, hair color, gender and IQ score). It also includes items learned by a person about herself from personal experiences or by internalizing the judgments of others.[2]

> *The voice in your head is constantly analyzing and interpreting distressful moments in an attempt to protect you from any situation that resembles your past traumas.*

This mental picture, or self-image, attaches itself to your doubts and fears and seeks to confirm its validity by connecting current and past experiences that evoke similar emotional responses. Ultimately, your self-image creates a definitive perspective about your environment, yourself and your world.

Delusional Diva: Inner Dialogue about Your Appearance

This definitive perspective turns into a never-ending mental dialogue that I affectionately call your "Delusional Diva." Your Delusional Diva unconsciously runs the show. The Diva's mutterings may be positive and affirming; however, they are often nasty and oppressive. Your Delusional Diva may validate narcissistic behavior, condemn people who threaten you, drive you to obsession or belittle you into resignation.

The voice in your head is constantly analyzing and interpreting distressful moments in an attempt to protect you from any situation that resembles your past traumas. Though studies show that the media, the beauty establishment and the appearance-obsessed culture adversely affect women's self-esteem, these are not the culprits that ultimately destroy your spiritual beauty. Your Delusional Diva, the little voice in the back of your head, is the true saboteur of your self-image.

Do you ever stop and listen to that little voice in your head? Do you take the time to understand what it is trying to tell you and why? More than likely, your voice already told you what it thought about that question. Actually, it *never* stops telling you what it thinks!

Consider the following scenario in which my friend Rita found herself:

Rita finds a neighboring business's mail mixed in with hers. She has not had the chance to introduce herself and her company to this new business, so she decides to deliver their mail, in person, with some information about her company. When she walks into their office, she finds everyone dressed in button-up shirts, dark suits and closed-toe shoes. Because she is wearing a yellow, low-cut, v-neck dress with bold flower prints and stylish open-toe sandals, the moment she steps through the door, all eyes are on her.

This situation is not uncommon. A number of clients and friends have described just such a scenario. Each person responds differently based on her self-image. Here are just a few of the responses I have heard:

- "I am such a fool! Why do I *always* wear the wrong thing at the wrong time?"

- "This is so *embarrassing*! Why didn't anyone tell me the dress code?"

- "Oh, well. It never fails. I *never* fit in. I guess I won't tell them how great my company is."

- "Ah, it's great to be the center of attention. I should go back again and drop off more literature."

Many dismiss this voice as a random rambling of the mind. However, if you analyze your Delusional Diva's babbling, you will be surprised by how dominant her voice is, and you may finally realize how greatly it affects the person you have become.

Beauty Characters Emerge from Your Delusional Diva's Dialogue

Your inner dialogue analyzes the world around you and justifies how you act in that world, even when your actions do not serve your happiness. The voice in your head molds you into what I call "Beauty Characters." Each of these Beauty Characters explained on the following pages exhibits different behavioral patterns, including distinct strategies to deal with your appearance, self-perception and worldview.

Throughout the years, I have observed and identified seven beauty-related characters that women play. These roles—and the behaviors connected to them—are a person's attempt to deal with her lack of acceptance and restore her sense of wholeness. These coping mechanisms exist for women whether they consider themselves ravishing, beautiful, pretty or plain.

Women develop Beauty Characters after an event in their life gives them a clue as to whether they are accepted or acceptable. The Beauty Characters, often adopted at a very young age, continue to morph and expand throughout adolescence, teenage years and young adulthood.

Some women adopt different aspects of each character or blend multiple characters in their entirety into a singular character. In this case, no single character is better than the other one. All Beauty Characters, in their own way, lead a person to strive for a sense of acceptance, validation and wholeness. Women may also use these characters to conceal or cope with rejection.

The concept of Beauty Characters should give you some insight into how you subconsciously respond when it comes to your appearance. Use it as a tool to become more self-aware, not as another label to place on yourself. If you are able to identify with any of these characters and their behaviors, it will help you to identify instances in which you are reacting subconsciously and in turn enable you to make different choices.

Each of these behaviors provides some form of relief from feeling as if your current circumstances control you. They are automatic ways of being that keep us from tackling the underlying issues that created each of the Beauty Characters in the first place.

Here is a description of each Beauty Character and its usual mode of operation. See if you, or someone you know, fit into one or more of these categories.

The Beauty Aficionado

She is a devotee and enthusiast of beauty, with an affinity for aesthetics. She loves experimenting with products and styles. Looking great and putting effort into her appearance are redeeming pursuits and are usually fun social activities for an Aficionado. Putting her looks on display for people to notice gives her the self-gratification and reassurance for which her Delusional Diva is looking. This exhibitive behavior is not isolated to her appearance. Her relationships, career and home also play a part. That look and pause in her conversation are the prompts to praise her new boyfriend, hair treatment or promotion. If someone denies an Aficionado the attention she desires, she may go to great lengths to make sure she gets her due recognition.

The Beauty Addict

She is obsessed with beauty products and procedures that will improve her looks, trying in vain to satisfy unrealistic standards or quell fears about the approval of others. An Addict works hard to cover up her insecurities. She commonly turns to makeup, procedures, excessive clothing or the lack thereof as her solution to this constant struggle. She may have a mild fixation, such as regular Botox, or go to extreme lengths with potentially damaging cosmetic procedures. Regardless, she feels that the rewards of acceptance far outweigh the risks. Her judgments about her appearance are harsh, and she will never give up trying to convince the person in the mirror that something about her needs fixing. A Beauty Addict desperately wants to fit in and will do whatever it takes to fix what she feels is not right with her life.

The Beauty Authority

She is convinced that she is an expert on beauty and is determined to have the goods to prove it. She tends to be a trendsetter and judges others from a position of superiority. She has confidence in her grasp of aesthetics and appearances. An Authority may turn into an ice queen, fashioning her appearance into a suit of armor that fends off anyone who does not compliment her style. An Authority maintains impeccable exterior style and grace to keep up with the high standards of her career, creativity, relationships or social status. Others may have teased her, or she may have failed badly at an early age. Her actions result from her fear of others' judgment.

The Beauty Amateur

She can dabble or put excessive effort into enhancing her appearance, but she is rarely—if ever—satisfied with the outcome. Deep down, she wishes that she could be as uninhibited and confident as an Aficionado or an Authority in her expression of beauty. The Amateur will buy clothes and leave them to die in her closet because she doubts that they could ever look as good on her as they did in the store or magazine. No matter how much time or money she spends on her clothes, makeup, hair and figure, it always seems to come out wrong. She beats herself up for not knowing exactly what to do. While growing up, an Amateur may have lacked acknowledgment or felt put down in comparison to her peers. She is stuck in her fashion pitfalls because she does not want to expose her vulnerabilities by asking for guidance.

The Beauty Dropout

She feels hopeless about her appearance and has a resigned, self-deprecating attitude toward her beauty. She puts more effort into putting herself down than she puts into improving her looks, and she wishes that she could trade in what she has to work with and start over as someone else. Her Delusional Diva taunts her with whispers of, "Why even try to improve your looks or update that 80's hairstyle? You should have contempt for your appearance and for your unique features." The Dropout always has an excuse to go home early or not go out at all. The less people see her, the safer she feels. Someone could have embarrassed her as a child for her appearance. Her Delusional Diva uses that moment as a reason to whisper, "Why bother? No one likes you anyway."

The Beauty Evader

She is indifferent or sometimes disdainful toward the value of appearances and beauty. She declines to put effort into enhancing her appearance and dedicates her energy to a career or hobbies that tend to be traditionally unfeminine. One would never catch her at a cosmetics counter or in a salon for anything more than a haircut. An Evader typically dresses in unflattering, drab clothing, which may be excessively work- or hobby-related, genderless in style or ill fitting. She may rarely update her wardrobe or take those extra steps to care for her body. If she does, it is more for health or recreation purposes than to elevate her beauty. Sometimes, an Evader neglects caring for aspects of her physical appearance or personal hygiene. She hides behind her ordinary style to dissuade others from paying attention to her looks. The Evader wants to be valued for her innate abilities or qualities, but she may secretly wish the same for her physical appearance. She will never admit it, however.

For the majority of my life, I played the role of a Beauty Evader, dressing more for form than for style or the attention of others. I wanted recognition for what I could do and how much I achieved—not the way I looked. Although I always cared for my well-being and hygiene, I avoided wearing makeup until I was well out of college. Of course, this drove my mother (the blossoming Mary Kay beauty consultant) crazy!

The Beauty Rebel

She opposes the popular beauty establishment and bitterly views most expressions of beauty as a superficial undermining of her womanhood. Punk rockers, hippies and avant-garde types may revel in nonconforming looks, which demonstrates their insurgence against common beauty standards. In a fit of resentful teen angst, or as part of an intellectualized statement-making agenda, Rebels love to make their opposition known. Fashion choices can stem from their unique experiences and modes of self-expression. A Rebel's defiance avoids values of conformity to which they do not measure up or which remind them of inferior or oppressive past experiences. The fifth piercing on her upper lip could be inspired self-expression or a way to defy society's standards for beauty. As with all Beauty Characters, a Rebel's Herstory is fundamental to understanding the inner dialogue behind her actions.

Exercise: Determine Your Beauty Character and Its Effect on You

As I said before, please use the concept of Beauty Characters only as a means to become more aware of how you automatically behave when it comes to your appearance. As the book continues, I will give you more tools to help you break free from operating on autopilot. You will become capable of creating an authentic expression of beauty that is in alignment with your beliefs about beauty.

- **Location:** A quiet place where you will not be disturbed

- **Materials:** Journal or paper, pen or pencil and a timer

- **Set your timer for:** 20–30 minutes of uninterrupted time

- **Preparation:** Take five minutes to go within and quiet your mind.

- **Instructions:** Read about the different Beauty Characters in this chapter, and choose the one that sounds like you. You are likely to find yourself in more than one character. For the purpose of this exercise, however, choose only one. Once you have identified your Beauty Character, write down your responses to the following questions with as much transparency as possible:

- What Beauty Character do you currently portray?

- What Beauty Characters did you play at different stages of your life (include your age for each one)?

- What behavioral patterns and strategies did you use at different times in your life?

- How did those behavioral patterns and strategies affect your life choices? Relationships? Career? Finances?

- What else does your Delusional Diva consistently tell you about yourself? About life? About others? About your past? About your future?

- How does your Delusional Diva's commentary affect your daily actions and choices?

- Who was directly involved when your Herstory occurred? What was their role?

- Who else did your Herstory affect? How did it affect them?

- Who has your Beauty Character affected? In what ways?

- Do your behavioral patterns and strategies have a positive or negative effect on you? On others?

- How have these reoccurring patterns or strategies affected your relationships? Career? Social life? Romantic relationships? The way you manage your money?

- What feelings are evoked by identifying these behaviors and the results they have produced?

Can you see how your past and your inner voice have shaped your behavior toward your appearance? If you don't see consistent patterns or behaviors, do not worry. Move on to the next chapter. As you advance through the next few chapters and encounter other women's stories, the impact of your inner voice may become more evident.

Do not let your Delusional Diva get you down. The point of this exercise is to make you aware of what could be limiting you or what could be standing in the way of your full self-expression. Awareness will enable you to break free from your burdening patterns and make choices that will uplift you in your quest for Fearless Beauty!

Awareness will enable you to break free from your burdening patterns and make choices that will uplift you in your quest for Fearless Beauty!

CHAPTER 3

Revealing Reflections— How the Past Shapes Who You See in the Mirror Every Day

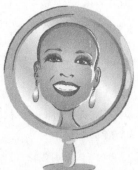

The beauty of a woman must be seen from in her eyes, because that is the doorway to her heart, the place where love resides.

—Audrey Hepburn

My Herstory: The Pink Cadillac

My Herstory begins at age five. I am riding in the backseat of my father's 1979 pink Cadillac Coupe de Ville; my father is driving and my mom is sitting in the front seat next to him. The sun is shining over Chicago, and we are on our way to my aunt's house for my cousin's birthday celebration. Music flows from the radio, and I am as happy as can be, looking out the window and counting houses.

The car rolls up to a stoplight and my eyes go wide. I sit up and shout with great joy.

"Daddy, that's *Rachel's* house!"

Those four words open Pandora's Box. Shock falls over my mom's face. Tears fall from her eyes, and she begins to slap my father uncontrollably. I think that Rachel is just a friend of the family that I have visited with my dad on numerous occasions; I have no clue that she is actually my dad's mistress.

My dad swerves the car to the side of the road and tries, unsuccessfully, to calm my mother down. Before I know it, they are both in a rage, screaming incoherently at each other. I sit in the backseat, crying at the top of my lungs and begging them to stop. It is a horrible scene, unlike any I have witnessed between them. I feel as if either might do something to fatally hurt the other.

A police officer arrives out of nowhere to settle them down, and once he leaves, my father resumes driving as if everything is back to normal. After this day, however, everything will be far from normal.

In this moment, my five-year-old self determines that what comes out of my mouth causes people to fight. I make a vow that I will keep religiously for the next 16 years: I do not speak to most people unless they speak to me—unless I am certain that my answer will not cause any pain. I vow to muzzle my self-expression. At five years old, my confidence is shattered.

My parents remained married and raised me in the same household; however, my relationship with my dad grew distant and cold. I was too petrified to interact with him. He was ashamed by what had happened and afraid that I would get him in hot water again.

As I grew older, we would go days, and eventually weeks, without speaking. I remember moments at the dinner table when I asked my mother to ask "her husband" to pass the ketchup. At times, I would beg my mom not to involve my dad in family events, such as my birthday, family reunions or vacations. I held such contempt for my father that I could not see how unbelievably nasty and hurtful I was acting. My trust in my father was broken. My Delusional Diva insisted I protect myself from further pain. Thus, I remained constantly on guard around my father.

The Backpack Kid

Before that drive-by at Rachel's house, I was close with both of my parents. Moreover, my dad and I were like peanut butter and jelly. Whenever my dad wasn't working, we spent a lot of time together. Everyone affectionately called me the "backpack kid" because everywhere he went, I was hanging on his back instead of buckled in a stroller.

On that fateful day, however, my relationship with my dad changed. It felt as if my dad's love for me had disappeared. I was no longer the backpack kid. I did everything to hide it, but I craved affection from my father to make me feel lovable, accepted and worthy again.

The aftermath of this altered relationship also inhibited how I navigated through my life, related to others and twisted my self-perception. When someone said, "Oh, Kenetia, you're so pretty!" I would think, "Well, you say that now. If you *really* knew me, though, you would leave me because my words cause pain."

The pain I thought I caused between my parents did not allow me to recognize my beauty, regardless of how many people complimented me. Though I didn't realize it, the love withheld from me and my own feelings of disdain directed toward my father made me feel ugly on the inside. Ultimately, ugly is how I viewed myself. I thought, "I *must* be unlovable because my dad shunned me. Others will surely abandon me, just as he did."

I distorted my self-perception. I believed that I looked unpleasant because of how I felt on the inside. I actively pushed my dad away—and many others close to me—out of fear that they would reject me.

Many women whom I have known, personally and professionally, have shared their stories about how their childhood traumas are constant reminders of their inability to see their beauty and capabilities. Janice, a client of mine who had me do her makeup regularly, revealed that her mother called her ugly when she was only seven years old. She also recalled her mother telling her that if she didn't find a way to be more pleasing, she would never amount to anything. Though Janice is now married, raises two beautiful children and works as a successful attorney, her Delusional Diva still tells her that she is ugly. She believes nothing she does is good enough, although everything she does is near-perfect. She often finds herself tired from all her efforts to prove that she is worthy of being loved.

My friend Shannon, who moved from California to New York at the age of six, is another example of how a woman's Herstory can haunt her. Shannon remembers the kids in her school teasing her because she was biracial (her mom is black and her father is white). She has an angelic spirit, but she will not speak up or follow her passion to teach because she is terrified of ridicule.

In reading this book, you may realize that something from your past makes you feel a bit modest about your appearance. It might also hinder you from doing what you are most passionate about in life. On the other hand, you might find that you overcompensate to prove to yourself and others that your past wrongs were unjust. Your Herstory can reach quite deep and very wide.

Turning Myself Inside Out

For years, I turned myself inside out to hide my longing for my dad's affection. The way I styled my hair, the fancy clothing I wore and my incessant, attention-seeking desire to succeed were all parts of my strategy to compensate for the loss of my father's acceptance and love.

Although the scenery, people and times changed, I kept reliving my Herstory.

Having that heartbreak constantly replay in my subconscious directly affected my behavior, my relationships, my self-image and, later, my career. Although the scenery, people and times changed, I kept reliving my Herstory. I constantly felt insecure, and I felt crushed when anyone broke up with me. I also gave up on relationships preemptively, assuming the love would disappear eventually anyway.

Uncovering my Herstory took courage and willingness to face my upsetting past. It was an emotional ride, but not all of it was painful. It was also a cathartic exploration, which led me to be at peace with the person in the mirror.

If you are willing to look deeply into your Herstory, you will begin to see what distorts the lens through which you view your self-image. This is the first step to unleashing your genuine expression of beauty.

> *If you are willing to look deeply into your Herstory, you will begin to see what distorts the lens through which you view your self-image.*

Start with the Truth

To get to the heart of your Herstory, start by being honest about what you tell yourself every time you step in front of the mirror. It takes courage to be forthright about all of those stories and assessments swarming around in your brain.

This exercise can be challenging, but the result is worth it. You will need deep-down dirty honesty to make it work, as well as the highest dose of compassion you can muster. Do not beat yourself up for beating yourself up!

Exercise: Use the Mirror

As you go through the steps of this exercise, remember to notice what goes through your mind, and make notes of exactly what you observe. Then, let it be. If your thoughts or emotions seem to take off running, just observe the nature of what you think and feel. Write that down as well.

- Location: A quiet place where you will not be disturbed
- Materials: A full-length mirror, a pad of paper or your journal, something to write with and a timer
- Set your timer for: 60–90 minutes of uninterrupted time
- Preparation: Take five minutes to go within and quiet your mind.

- **Instructions:** Stand or sit in front of your mirror (whichever is more comfortable). Set your timer for two minutes and look at the person in the mirror for the full two minutes. I promise she won't jump out at you or hurt you in any way! Do a full body scan, starting at your head and moving down the rest of your body. Focus on one area at a time.

Once your timer sounds at two minutes, take the next 10 to 20 minutes to write down every thought you can capture that popped into your mind about your appearance within those two minutes.

After you have written down your thoughts, ask yourself the following questions and write down your answers. It may help to close your eyes, take a few deep breaths and pause to digest what you see before moving to the next question.

- What was your experience of being in front of the mirror looking at yourself?

- Describe the person you see in the mirror.

- What do you like or dislike about this person? Do you see anything praiseworthy or flawed?

- Using the words in the below list (only if they apply), write down the words that best describe how you feel about your appearance. What words are not listed that would also describe how you feel about your appearance?

relaxed	confident	frantic	happy	attractive
weak	dull	sexy	disgusted	feminine
scared	gorgeous	tired	anxious	uncomfortable
natural	ugly	cute	unhealthy	uninterested
fit	rigid	pretty	average	sophisticated

- Describe the emotions around any positive or negative commentary that you feel about particular parts of your body. For example:

  - "When I look at my forehead, it reminds me of my mom, and I feel bitter."

  - "I love my lips. They are full and kissable."

  - "I feel embarrassed by my teeth and want to replace them."

  - "My eyes have a sultry sparkle and make me feel confident because they draw people in."

  - "My weight is normal, but I do not like how I carry it. I feel awkward in tight clothing."

Are you hearing these comments, feelings and assessments for the first time? These thoughts—or some version closely resembling them—are by-products of your Herstory and evidenced in the criticism uttered by your Delusional Diva. They have been intruding on you and affecting your life for years.

Examine what you experienced and wrote down during the mirror exercise to distinguish elements of your Herstory. Parts of your Herstory may remain hidden from you after this particular exercise, but as you continue with the next exercise, more will surface.

Exercise: How Has the Past Shaped You?

"Behavioral scientists say that, by the age of two, 50% of what people believe about themselves has been formed; by age six, 60% of self-belief has been established; by age eight, almost 80%. By the age of 14, over 99% have a well-developed sense of whom and what they believe themselves to be."[1]

It is important to understand that most of the things you believe to be true about yourself were formed at a very early age. Your Delusional Diva serves as a filter that you perceive all of your life experiences through, including the imagery and media that you consume. Until you address the meaning you have assigned to yourself based on the events of your past, it is extremely difficult to view yourself objectively. When women hit 20, their Delusional Diva has them locked in her grasp, imposing consistent justification for their vanity or reinforcing disapproval or numbness toward her appearance. The damaging consequences of my Herstory, and my Diva's strategy to deal with it, were at the root of the way my whole life progressed, from childhood through adulthood.

Read through everything you have written about your appearance, and think back to the earliest time in your life when you can remember having these views of yourself. It will not be last week, so keep going back in two- to four-year increments to see if those thoughts existed before today.

Scan your memory until you get to an earlier age when you may not have had the words to express how you were feeling, but you knew that something was wrong and it didn't feel good.

Write out what happened in simple language. If possible, express how the little girl who experienced the past event, or events, would have expressed it using the language that she would have used. The idea is to express your emotional experiences on paper. If your recollection seems unclear, do not stress out about getting your stories exactly right. Just keep thinking about them.

You can also approach this in reverse if your memories are foggy. Recall a time in your young life when you *did not* feel there was anything wrong at all. Life was good and everything was perfect. Then, something happened that burst your idyllic bubble, broke your heart, upset you or stung your ego for the first time.

Maybe you were merely an observer in this event. Maybe one of your parents left home, a friend got into a serious accident or your younger sister was born.

Here are some questions to help you remember:

What is your earliest memory of feeling this emotion?

*Event #1:*_____

_____

*Event #2:*_____

_____

*Event #3:*_____

_____

How old were you when you first had these thoughts about yourself?

*Event #1:*_____

_____

*Event #2:*_____

_____

*Event #3:*_____

_____

Where were you?

*Event #1:*_____

_____

*Event #2:*_____

_____

*Event #3:*_____

_____

What were you doing?

Event #1: _____

_____

Event #2: _____

_____

Event #3: _____

_____

Who was around?

Event #1: _____

_____

Event #2: _____

_____

Event #3: _____

_____

What was said?

Event #1: _____

_____

Event #2: _____

_____

Event #3: _____

_____

Describe, in detail, what happened.

*Event #1:*_____

_____

*Event #2:*_____

_____

*Event #3:*_____

_____

You may start to notice multiple events in your past that affected you this way. Beginning with the earliest one, complete this chapter's exercise. Then, go back and complete the exercise for as many past events as you like.

Once you have completely described the event in detail, you will see how this episode began to dictate your future and shape how you view yourself. What did you tell yourself or decide about your life when all this happened?

Do any of the following statements resound with what you decided in that moment?

- "There is something wrong with me."

- "I must be bad," ". . . great," ". . . ugly," or ". . . beautiful."

- "I am stupid."

- "They (or people) are stupid."

- "What's wrong with everyone?"

- "I will not let that happen again."

- "I am not lovable. / They don't love me. / No one cares."

- "I am not good enough. / They are better than I am."

- "I'll show them that I am good enough (or better than they are)."

- "People are scary. / People can hurt you."

- "I don't care anymore."

Start to connect the dots between your Herstory and the inner dialogue you noted while doing the mirror exercise. Because you were young, it was simply natural to interpret the events around you and accept that interpretation as an accurate explanation of those events. Once you accepted that interpretation as fact, it had a lingering effect on your self-worth and your identity.

For example, if you experienced people as scary when you were young, chances are that you became a shy, withdrawn person to avoid feeling afraid. Perhaps you became an icy, mean person to combat your fear of people. Perhaps you avoided them altogether. Even if you see yourself as beautiful and happy, you may notice that your Herstory has limited or even suffocated your fullest expression of beauty, your communication skills or your behavior.

If you can release yourself from the confines of even one of the judgments from your past, you will feel more at ease about the person you face every time you look in the mirror. Then you can begin to awaken the extraordinarily beautiful being you really want to see in your reflection.

Please feel free to revisit this exercise whenever you recall other past events that have had a deep effect on you. Also, return to this exercise if the mirror starts acting up again and has nasty things to say about you.

CHAPTER 4

The Delusional Diva's Demise— Release the Pain That Binds You to Your Fears

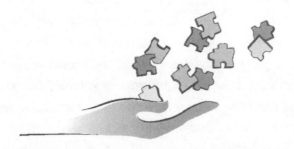

The interpretation of our reality through patterns not our own, serves only to make us ever more unknown, ever less free, ever more solitary.

—Gabriel Garcia Márquez

How Does Your Delusional Diva Affect Your Subconscious Thoughts?

The entire construction of your Herstory is not about what actually happened in your past but rather your *interpretation* of what happened. I am not implying that those events did not actually occur. They did. However, allowing things said about you, by others or yourself, to define you is a decision you made on your own. Allowing that definition to dictate your life from that day forward is also a decision you made.

Your Delusional Diva uses your Herstory to identify potential threats in your life. It matches

Your Diva uses whatever strategy works best, even if it means sabotaging things you really want.

those threats with experiences from your past, and then acts to protect you. Your Diva uses whatever strategy works best, even if it means sabotaging things you really want.

For example, you may desire to receive compliments for how well you look in a dress you just purchased. Then, the moment your boyfriend opens his mouth to say, "Oh honey, you look sexy in that dress," you shut him down or assume he didn't mean it. This scenario plays out because your Delusional Diva controls your subconscious. When it tells you that nothing you do will ever inspire anyone to notice you, you act in a way that confirms its statements.

The nonstop chatter in your head, which follows you everywhere, subliminally tells you how to avoid further heartbreak. Your Diva's devious, scheming behavior roots deeply into your subconscious, and you become submerged in it. Because you become accustomed to hearing her talk, you stop consciously paying attention to her. Like water to a fish or air to a bird, your Diva's talk engulfs you all the time and fades into the backdrop of life. You no longer realize it even exists.

When your mind registers something common to you—such as seeing the same sights on your drive to work every day—you overlook the details. The same is true for your Herstory and the voice in your head that results. Although unnoticed, they relentlessly define your behavior and self-image.

How Did My Delusional Diva Affect My Behavior?

I grew up unaware of the extent to which the rift in the relationship with my dad affected my life. My fear of repeated rejection and my feelings of being unworthy were the water in the sea all around me. The loss of affinity for someone about whom I deeply cared, and my fear of growing close to others, swiftly brought my Delusional Diva into action. She barked the orders to build defenses. She then told me how to view what I saw in the mirror, how to "fix" what I saw, how to interpret what people said to me, and how to choose, distance myself from, and end relationships. All of these tactics were attempts to protect me from facing future rejection.

In the fourth grade, I asked my teacher if I could become an astronaut when I grew up. She told me that I could do anything I wanted to do if I just "put my pretty little head to it." On the surface, her comment sounded encouraging. Nevertheless, my nine-year-old brain sifted her kind words through the grid of my Herstory. I shaped her comment into something malicious.

What I "heard" was that I needed to work hard if I was going to do well at anything because I did not have the smarts to make it. "Pretty" was something I often heard from people when I was young. However, the voice in my head told me that their compliments were undeserved because I did not have the love and approval from the one person who really mattered—my dad.

When I heard these types of compliments, I would think, "Oh, they're just trying to be nice. If they *really* knew me, like my dad does, they wouldn't like me either."

I thought that being "pretty" meant that my looks were all I had, and I needed to compensate for that fact. This was the insecure thinking of a fourth grader, a self-assessment consistent with the one I made when I was five. In addition to feeling unworthy of love, I believed that I needed to try harder to accomplish anything because I was merely "pretty."

My Delusional Diva kept me searching for proof that I must not be good enough—that I was unlovable—so she could defend me when that proof showed up. I found evidence of this belief in my interpretation of experience, not in reality. I filtered everything through my belief that I was unworthy.

Deep down, I yearned for a substitute to replace the love and affection I was missing from my father, which was the source of my insecurities. Those feelings stewed inside of me and wrecked my confidence. So when my fourth-grade teacher made a comment that included the word "pretty," it hit right at the heart of my fading self-esteem.

My Diva snapped back in defense, "I'll show her and everyone else that I'm not *just* pretty. I can be good at everything!"

The strategy my Diva devised was winning—winning at board games, school elections, sports, or anything at which I could compete. The accolades would prove that I could be good enough at *something,* even if I could not win with my dad. These victories were the shaky foundation on which I built my life. My insecurities and fear of rejection, which my Diva desperately wanted to buffer out, were seeping into the cracks and would eventually bring the whole house down.

As I grew older, I worked harder and harder to prove that I was capable of *everything*—that I was not just another pretty face. In college, I was the poster child for participation: tennis team, resident advisor, Black Student Union and Omicron Delta Kappa National Leadership Honors Society. I pushed myself to take six courses per semester (four was the norm) in order to graduate in three years. I did all of this while holding a night job as a records clerk at the municipal police station.

Fresh out of college, I worked 70 hours a week as a district manager for three health clubs, a job which actually only required a 50-hour workweek. I was ranked #1 in everything—sales, member retention, cleanliness. You name it; I was on top.

During those years, I was often asked, "Why are you doing so much? Are you trying to drive yourself *crazy*?"

The answer was that I drove myself to prove that I was *good* and *smart* enough. I even tried to show up my dad. I wanted him to know that he had made a big mistake in pushing away his daughter.

My Diva was persistent in creating strategies for covering up what I perceived as my weak spots and in setting me up to win in life, even at the cost of intimacy and happiness. As a teenager, I hungered for close relationships yet dodged them by being distant and superficial. I was so afraid that if people *really knew me,* they would see how hurtful I could be and reject me the same way my dad did.

I would meet a boy and fall deeply in love. Then I would dump him, or I would become completely uninterested by the next week. I never hung out with just one group of people. Socializing with a variety of groups ensured that I would not have to get too close to anyone.

I camouflaged my beauty and femininity with plain, loose-fitting clothes to keep the contours of my body invisible. I refused to wear provocative outfits when most high-school girls were trying to show off their goods and get boys' attention. I wanted people to know me for dressing properly and looking sharp, like a winner.

I stayed involved with team sports and group activities. I wanted people to recognize my worthiness as they witnessed me rack up the points and take the lead on projects. I thought that numerous achievements and voracious ambition would hide my churning self-image from the world. I hoped that by focusing on activities, I could avoid the relational destiny my Diva predicted for me—certain rejection and failure with intimacy.

Boy, was I wrong about *that*!

How Did My Delusional Diva Affect My Relationships?

As a determined, vulnerable young woman, I continued my pursuit of validation in a relationship that was a total inversion of the one I had with my father.

On a drizzly day—December 31, 1999—against a majestic Maui backdrop, I said, "I do." I was 23 years old and the groom was a man whom I had dated for five years. I loved him and knew he loved me. I found a supportive, no-nonsense guy whose whole mentality revolved around being smart. He was quite successful at everything he did.

He was handsome—without a playboy charisma—and a bit unassuming. I felt these qualities made him a safe bet and nullified any chance of his infidelity. He was a perfect complement to my entire agenda at the time. Moreover, I had chosen a mate who was the polar opposite of my dad: educated, studious, virtuous and by the book. We were best friends, and people often mistook our playful nature for that of a brother and sister.

I truly believed that I found a man who could be my partner. I finally felt as if I was a part of a relationship that was not predestined to fail. There was little to no chemistry or affection between us, and his asexual love for me was perfect. I believed that I wanted a man who loved me "for me" and not for my physical attributes. I thought my marriage to him proved that I was worthy, smart enough and more than "just another pretty face."

My marriage became another big victory for me, and I began to overlook what would have actually made it succeed. We communicated well with each other but never on a heartfelt level. We had a playmate type of friendship and laughed a lot, but there was little intimacy. We shared no deep connection. I don't believe that he felt safe enough to open up and be vulnerable with me, mainly because I was so driven and focused on myself at the time.

Our sex life quickly became nonexistent. This triggered my feelings of being unappreciated and undesirable. I tolerated it because of our amazing friendship though. The lack of physical attention made me question my femininity. I was constantly wondering what was wrong with me, and my self-esteem took another beating. I would look in the mirror and wonder, "Am I *ugly* now? Am I not *sexy* anymore?" After all these years working so hard to prove that I was more than just "pretty," here I was for the first time faced with feelings of being unattractive. I had no clue how to handle it.

I knew others felt that I was beautiful growing up, but I chose to discount my appearance and put greater importance on other things, such as my achievements. My Diva needed to figure out what to do about the reflection of the unfamiliar woman who was now staring back at me.

I was a novice at romance and intimacy, as was my husband—considering his lack of enthusiasm in the bedroom. We went to counseling, but he never did anything that the counselor recommended. My pleas for him to open up turned to nagging, then to rage, and then to complete resignation. It felt useless.

I began to wonder what else might be "out there," since my husband was not willing to explore sexual intimacy with me. After more than three years of marriage and nine months of unwanted celibacy, I broke my vows and cheated on my husband.

This new man gave me the appreciation for which I had been yearning while with my husband, but my feelings and discontentment with the status quo were not a valid justification to do what I did. No matter how I spun it, I gave my word to be faithful to my husband, and I was not.

The honorable thing would have been to talk more about our situation or end our relationship before getting involved with anyone else; however, my Delusional Diva was tired of feeling unworthy and demanded affection.

Certain aspects of my bond with my husband made me feel validated, but I had been set up by my Herstory to spend my life with a man who did not desire me sexually, thus fulfilling the notion that I wasn't good enough. I had my husband's love, but I was still unworthy of his physical affection—just like with my dad. He was everything my father was not, yet I was again craving intimacy. I had tricked myself into thinking this was not important.

Cheating on my husband did not resolve my negative feelings about myself. Every time I looked in the mirror, I felt ashamed. I was horrified that I was becoming more and more like my father, the man who was disloyal to my mother.

Months after my affair, my husband and I found ourselves unpacking boxes after moving halfway across the country—from Chicago, Illinois, to Burbank, California. I buried my affair inside me and vowed to myself that I would not speak a word about it. I was hopeful that a fresh start with a new life in a new city would bridge the rift between us.

Three months after our move to California, I entered our home and felt a chill rush through me. The house felt empty and cold.

"Hey, babe," I yelled. "Are you home?"

There was no reply.

I peeked in the bathroom and my husband was sitting there, his face full of dismay. Without knowing what was going on, my heart sank to my stomach. He told me that he found an email from the man with whom I had an affair. My husband proceeded to interrogate me about him. I denied everything, yet I could not bear the sadness in his eyes or his shattered heart. I finally told him that I had spent time with this man, but I did not confess anything more.

"God forbid," I thought. "We could end up in a hostile fight, and I could turn out to be the bad guy, just like my father."

I defended my actions by saying that this other man had shown me the attention that my husband had failed to give me for nine months.

"What were you doing to occupy *your* time?" I demanded.

What he told me broke my heart. If you assume that he also cheated on me, you are wrong. What he shared shook me to the core, but it is not for me to advertise.

We both lamented the shame of what had transpired. When he opened up to me, I felt compassion and empathy for my husband rather than justification or bitterness. We ended the conversation by forgiving each other and promising that we would do right by each other going forward. It felt as if we had a renewed relationship.

One year later, we were back in the same rut. We were two asexual organisms once again, and although I felt the distance weighing on me, I was clear that I was not going to stray. I wanted the kind of lasting relationship that we both felt our parents had.

The morning of my birthday, I awoke to a typical, sunny Southern California day. Temperatures were in the low 80s, and the scenery was right out of a Hollywood movie. The streets were lined with palm trees; the sky was crystal clear. My husband and I walked to our favorite diner for breakfast. After we ate, we sat in silence.

He cleared his throat and spoke.

"I'm not happy."

"Okay. What do you want to do about it?"

His aloof response shocked me.

"Nothing."

"What do you mean *nothing*? Don't you want to get counseling? What do you want me to do while you're not happy?"

Tears streamed down my face. I felt embarrassed and hurt, considering that I would have done anything to make sure we worked it out. Clearly, that was not his plan.

I stared deeply into his eyes in complete silence. My sorrow quickly turned into anger. I got up, left the table and marched back to our home alone. Before I reached the front door, I knew in my heart that there was no way I could withstand another month without intimacy.

After seven years of what I thought was a good marriage, I packed up a few possessions and moved to a tiny studio 40 minutes away from my husband and right across the street from my new job with L'Oreal Paris.

At the end of an exhausting day of moving into my new home, I knew it was time to call my mother to tell her that I had left my husband. It was the one call I really dreaded. I believed in my heart that, regardless of my reason for leaving, she would feel that it was not sensible. Despite years of trying to prove that I was winning in my life, I was certain that my mom would view this as a major failure. I was prepared for her to write me off as a huge disappointment.

I called and told her a few details. She was confused.

"Where did you two move to?"

"No, Mom. *I* moved."

"What do you mean?" she replied, with heavy concern in her voice.

"Well, I packed up my things and moved into a studio apartment not far from work."

"Why would you do *that*? Are you separating from your husband?" The storm cloud burst, and the questions rained down. "Why? What *happened*? How come you didn't tell me about this *before*?" Then, the words I dreaded shot out of her mouth: "I am *definitely* disappointed and really sad, but are *you* okay?"

I did not want to respond, but I managed to say a few words.

"I'm doing fine, but I gotta go. I need to prepare for work tomorrow. We can talk about this another time."

We hung up the phone, and I burst into tears. My mother endured so much in order to keep her marriage together with a man who was unfaithful to her. Here I was, after seven years of marriage, telling her that I was calling it quits.

The Full Circle

My Herstory carved a path for my life that had come full circle. I felt that I had disappointed my mother, just as my dad had done. My Delusional Diva drove me to avoid intimacy and potential rejection, and now I had arrived at my destination. This was the beginning of a total meltdown in my health, vitality and strength of mind. I felt help-less to stop it.

My fear of being unloved and unworthy permeated everything in my life, from becoming a self-centered achievement junkie (because my fourth-grade teacher called me "pretty") to blindly repressing my sexual needs (by marrying a man who had zero interest in real intimacy with me).

> *My Herstory carved a path for my life that had come full circle.*

I desperately wanted others to recognize me for more than my looks. I wanted to be valued for what I accomplished. My Delusional Diva turned this desire into frantic ambitions, which led to major breakdowns in every area of my life. Even though I desperately desired intimacy, I suppressed my self-expression in relationships with my parents and my husband. My self-esteem and eventually my entire well-being also took a beating. My Diva always sabotaged the things I wanted most in an effort to protect me.

The Fallout and Impact of Your Herstory

Your Herstory's development and the ways in which it affects your life may be similar or vastly different from my own. It may feel like a walk in the park, a roller-coaster ride through hell, or anywhere in between. Regardless of your experience with your Herstory, the Delusional Diva that grows from it may be denying what you truly want in life every time she opens her mouth.

The longer you wait to address how your past and inner voice affect your behavior, the more you may tolerate being unsatisfied with your life and, subsequently, your physical appearance. Confronting the inner workings of your Delusional Diva and the impact the past has had on your life is an opportunity to discover those oppressive patterns that prevent you from being truly

Confronting the inner workings of your Delusional Diva and the impact the past has had on your life is an opportunity to discover those oppressive patterns that prevent you from being truly happy.

happy. This will help you identify the Beauty Character you have adopted and remove the limitations that accompany it. Until you break free from these constructs and limitations, your Delusional Diva will continue to work hard to protect you from being hurt.

Repetition is the simplest formula for keeping yourself afloat. Your Diva goes to extremes to search for potential threats. She protects you from threats, using whatever method is effective. Once a strategy works (as winning did for me), you will replicate it until that strategy breaks down—or you break down from all of the strategizing.

Why is your Diva so unreliable at making your life simple and enjoyable? Your Diva usually appears at such a young age that you do not yet have the vocabulary or the emotional intelligence to understand your need to defend against experiences that you do not like. In your young mind, you know that you do not like what has happened. Then you interpret it to mean that there is something wrong with you, with other people or with the world.

My Diva galloped in to protect me after that first heartbreak in the car in front of Rachel's house. I was only five years old. I made up my Herstory to avoid my dad and to avoid being close to people because rejection was too much to bear in the mind of such a young a child.

At the impressionable age of five, my Diva was running my life. It was already exhausting me! There is no fulfillment or joy in a life built around efforts to break free from feelings of inadequacy. You may often filter your perception of life through the emotional sensibility of a young child who is still seeking validation or trying to avoid pain. The saddest part is, because I was unconscious of the merry-go-round on which I sat, I could do nothing to stop the ride.

My inner voice loves to issue the warning, "Back off. Don't get too close or try to reject me . . . or I'll show you that I don't need you. I'm a *winner!*"

These types of subliminal, knee-jerk reactions are severely limiting. They prevent you from your full self-expression. It does not matter if you are a business tycoon, a drama queen, a happily married woman or a man-eater. Your nature is one of repeating patterns of success, crisis, comfort, insecurity, illness, unpredictability, sexual prowess, dormancy, restlessness or whatever mode of operation your Beauty Character dictates.

By recognizing that your past is running the show, you can choose to let it go or remain with the effects of what you made up about yourself at that very young age.

Exercise: Expand on Your Herstory as You Remember It

- **Location:** A quiet place where you will not be disturbed
- **Materials:** Your Herstory (see "Exercise: Use the Mirror" in Chapter 3), journal or paper, and a timer

- **Set your timer for:** 60–90 minutes of uninterrupted time

- **Preparation:** Take five minutes to go within and quiet your mind.

- **Instructions:** In detail, expand on what you wrote in the Chapter 3 exercise by describing the place, colors, smells and any sensations in order to capture the tone and emotions while the event occurred. Create the story as if it were a contender for an Academy Award for Best Picture! Write it out exactly as you remember it.

It is also important at this stage to capture all of the emotions and feelings you experienced before, during and after the event took place. If the event was traumatic, explain why you felt that it was traumatic. If the story was light and laughable, add humor.

Don't hold back . . . *tell your story!*

Exercise: Read Through Your Herstory

- **Location:** A quiet place where you will not be disturbed

- **Materials:** The revised, edited version of your Herstory from the previous exercise as well as a tissue, something soft and squeezable, a pillow, a comfy chair and a timer

- **Set your timer for:** 60–90 minutes of uninterrupted time

- **Preparation:** Take five minutes to go within and quiet your mind.

- **Instructions:** While sitting in your comfortable spot, with your tissue and something soft and squeezable and/or your pillow near you, read your Herstory aloud all the way through, word for word.

Do not be alarmed if a rush of emotions runs through you as you read your Herstory aloud. You may giggle, you may cry, or you may feel numb. Whatever emotions arise within you, do not suppress them. Just let them flow. The first time I read my Herstory, I could barely see through all the tears that were streaming down my face.

After you have read your Herstory aloud, take a deep breath and read it again from the beginning. Do not deviate from the story by adding something to it or taking something out. Just read it as you wrote it, word for word.

You may feel no differently than the first time you read it. You may feel more or less emotional. Again, breathe and let your emotions do what they do. Do not try to fix the way you are reacting to your story. Be in the moment, and go at your own pace. Avoid getting up or doing anything that distracts you from being present with your Herstory and your emotions.

Take a few more deep breaths. Then reread your Herstory three more times all the way through. If you still feel the same intensity of emotion that you experienced the first couple of times, read your Herstory again all the way through. If you started out feeling numb and your feelings are growing more intense as you read, you are doing great.

Keep reading your Herstory and be aware of your emotions. There is no need to react to them. Do not worry about whatever comes up for you; just experience those thoughts and emotions without judgment.

Exercise: Add Theatrics to Your Herstory

- **Location:** A quiet place where you will not be disturbed—one big enough to move around freely, if needed

- **Materials:** The revised, edited version of your Herstory, the actor in you and a timer

- **Set your timer for:** 60–90 minutes of uninterrupted time

- **Preparation:** Take five minutes to go within and quiet your mind.

- **Instructions:** It is now time to add some play to this exercise! This part could prove to be fun, especially if you are still upset. The purpose of this exercise is to free you up from the emotional pain that the past may have caused you.

Read your Herstory again in the following ways:

- In a child's voice, at the age when you remember this story beginning

- As if you were on a Broadway stage in front of an audience of 300 people (Give it all you've got. This is your chance to shine!)

- In the voice of a character who is robust, who has a sense of humor and who makes you laugh, such as Miss Piggy, Lady Gaga, Betty White, Tina Fey or Carol Burnett . . . Let it rip!

- As if you were an important public figure, hoping to be re-elected

- As if you were on trial for a crime for which you just admitted guilt and you are pleading for the jury to give you mercy

At this point, you are either very tired of hearing your own Herstory, or your perception of the significance about what happened has diminished. Perhaps you are starting to see that the Herstory you wrote is just that: a story! Just like the fairy tales with which I was obsessed as a child, reading my Herstory over and over revealed that it was merely a distorted interpretation of what happened.

What actually happened was, I said, "Hey, that's Rachel's house!"

My parents fought, I cried my little head off and then we drove to my cousin's house. My interpretation of this event was that I was unlovable, that my dad hated me afterward and that he was a scary man who wanted to hurt my mom and me.

This was not true!

My experience was real, but none of the rest actually happened.

It is my hope that you now see the distinction between what really happened in your past and what you made this story mean about you and your life. They are not the same; your interpretation of events is rarely the same as what actually happened.

Your Delusional Diva created an interpretation of your Herstory to protect you from experiencing those painful emotions again. Thus, if you made up your whole Herstory as a defense mechanism, your Herstory is not real—and none of what you made up about yourself is real either! They are simply your interpretations of the events.

Once you are able to accept that the story you made up is just a story, you will likely breathe a big sigh of relief. If you are at this point, take it to the next level and bring forgiveness to the people in your story. If you have not let go of the significance of your Herstory, revisit the previous exercise with a loving and supportive friend who is willing to sit with you and listen to you tell your story multiple times.

Be sure to let them know that they are there just to listen and not to make judgments or defend how you feel about your Herstory. This is not a simple exercise. It is normal to take some time to work on it.

Remember: We are building muscles, not looking for quick fixes.

CHAPTER 5

Mindful Makeovers— Heal the Past and Change Your Future

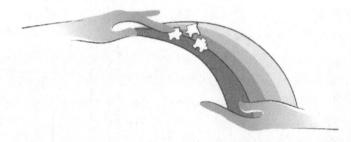

When you hold resentment toward another, you are bound to that person or condition by an emotional link that is stronger than steel. Forgiveness is the only way to dissolve that link and get free.

—Catherine Ponder

Courageous Acts of Forgiveness: Releasing My Herstory

On a cold winter night in Chicago, one unforgettable conversation changed my view of my dad and ultimately allowed me to see myself in a completely different light.

I was in my house hanging up the phone after attempting to dial my parents' number for the nineteenth time. Each time I got to the eighth digit, I hung up. I was trying to call my father after not speaking with him for over 15 years. My body was shaking, feverish sweat was pouring down my forehead and my heart was thumping so hard that I could see my sweater rising and falling on my chest.

On the twentieth try, my fingers dialed the number by accident and it rang. I hoped that no one would pick up, but then I heard my father's voice on the other end.

Everything in me said, "Hang up!" but other words came out instead.

"Hello, Dad. How are you?"

"Fine."

Without hesitation, he asked if I wanted to speak with my mother.

"No. Actually I called to speak with you."

I asked if he would allow me to speak without interruption, so I could say everything I needed to say.

He agreed.

I divulged every disgusting, icky, bitter, agonizing, remorseful sentiment onto which I had been holding for the past 15 years. Then I added a final declaration.

"I forgive you for what happened, Dad."

Something unspeakable came next. I asked him to forgive *me* for shutting him out and preventing him from being my dad.

> *My biggest fear became my greatest triumph in a matter of seconds.*

He was silent for what felt like an eternity. In the back of my mind, I thought that he was going to swear at me or just hang up. However, to my surprise, the most profound words came through the line.

"I love you, Kenetia."

I had never heard these words uttered from his mouth! Shock and relief overwhelmed my body. My biggest fear became my greatest triumph in a matter of seconds. For years, all I wanted was for us to be close again and love each other.

I got my dad back!

That conversation made me a believer in the power of forgiveness. For 15 years, I never spoke to him over the phone. He had never uttered the words "I love you" to my mother, at least not in front of me. Moreover, he had never said them to me.

My dad now calls me once a week to find out what I am up to, and he is usually more excited than I am to talk about it. And he never hangs up the phone without telling me that he loves me. Three years ago, I went home for an extended visit. It was the first time we ever went out for lunch alone and just enjoyed each other's company.

Forgiveness Brings Freedom

The shift in my relationship with my dad lifted a two-ton boulder off my back. I became less argumentative and more fun loving. I began to smile more and open up to people without feeling awkward or defensive. I communicated more clearly with people and became more at ease in relationships because of the newfound compassion that I felt for my dad. Now, I easily give up being righteous because I understand the cost of losing someone whom I dearly love.

I was incredibly hard on others, including myself, before I forgave my dad. I lived in protection mode, ready for my Diva to give the order that someone should be removed from my life because he or she did not deserve my attention. I was scared that friction from people was a sign that they were out to get me and that their rejection was looming. I would preemptively reject them to avoid the hurt of their dismissal.

I thought my dad was intentionally hurting my mom when he cheated on her. He later told me, "If I would have known better, I would have done better." It was a great relief to hear my dad voice his regret, and his sentiments were icing on the cake. My acceptance of him released me from the resentment I had been carrying around for more than 15 years. I could now see him as a human being instead of some evil monster.

I stopped viewing other people as the enemies as well. They could be my partners, and I could open up to them. I did not feel as if I needed to be someone I did not want to be. I could replace my defenses with compassion, peace of mind and love.

I felt freedom like never before!

Immediately after I forgave my father, I saw a shift in my marriage, even though it ended. I began to listen to my husband with greater compassion. When he spoke, I would patiently wait to hear everything he had to say before I responded. Before, I would cut him off mid-sentence, being far more interested in the earth-shattering importance of what *I* had to say than in listening to *him*.

I stopped worrying about what I wanted to get out of the relationship and began to understand the seriousness of my husband's situation. Opening up more of myself to him made me realize what I truly desired in my marriage. I began to uncover the inconsistencies between what my husband and I wanted out of life.

I had spent years riding the ups and downs of our marriage and attempting to work things out at all costs. As a result of my choice to extend forgiveness, my attitude was transformed, and I began to question why I felt as if I needed to stay in a relationship that was not fulfilling for either of us. I gradually learned to honor my feelings and identify what I wanted deep inside: a loving, affectionate relationship that fostered the appreciation of each other's beauty and self-expression. I stopped trying to hold on tightly to a marriage in which genuine compatibility did not exist. I no longer needed to prove my worth by forcing the marriage to succeed. Separating was a bold step out of the limitations of my Herstory toward an authentic new beginning.

Before taking that leap of faith and making the phone call to my father, I could not have imagined absolving him of guilt for the pain he had caused me. But I discovered that in choosing to forgive, I took back power that I didn't even know was lost. Forgiving what I previously felt was deplorable behavior helped me relax and let go of my defensiveness. It restored my faith in my dad as well as my ability to experience intimacy and connect with the human race. My heart was at ease. I was rid of resentment, blame, hurt and the idea that I was some sort of victim.

I discovered that in choosing to forgive, I took back power that I didn't even know was lost.

If releasing the emotional baggage from your past is not a compelling enough reason to offer forgiveness, it may help to realize some of the scientifically proven health benefits that forgiveness offers.

In a recent article entitled "Exploring Forgiveness," philosopher and renowned expert on forgiveness Joanna North asserts that forgiveness (when given or received) makes people healthier and happier. "Through forgiveness the pain and hurt caused by the original wrong are released, or at least they are not allowed to mar the whole of one's being for all time."[1]

I can personally attest to the physical benefits of releasing wrongs. After forgiving my father, my body fat decreased significantly, almost without any effort on my part, my posture straightened out, and my skin brightened up.

On the other hand, holding on to your reason for anger and resentment as if it were a precious deed of ownership is like holding on to a title to a polluted pond. Resisting forgiveness is toxic in how it affects your entire being.

The Mayo Clinic, a not-for-profit medical practice and research group, published a 2008 report that further detailed the ill effects of resentment. In their report, the Mayo Clinic found that people who held on to significant grudges showed increased blood pressure, heart rate, nicotine dependence and drug abuse. In addition, the study revealed that when people hold on to resentment, every subsequent relationship and experience may be marked by negativity or resignation.[2]

When people get riled up about offenses against them, they become stuck in their current mind state and/or emotions and cease to enjoy the present moment. Overwhelming resentment can lead to depression, anxiety, violent behavior and numbness. Anger and sadness can distance a person from other people and break precious connections. Some people may even feel that their lives lack inspiration, purpose or spirituality—as I did before forgiving my father.

Everett Worthington, Jr., a psychology professor at Virginia Commonwealth University, found that resentment triggers stress in the body, releasing high amounts of cortisol. Cortisol is a hormone produced by the adrenal glands that is responsible for inducing energy to fight stress reactions, regulate fat buildup in the body, and suppress inflammations. Excessive amounts of cortisol interfere with immune system function. This, in turn, weakens the body's ability to remain physically healthy and handle the mental and emotional stress with which a person may struggle. Holding on to resentment and blame clearly takes a spiraling toll on every aspect of a person's life, including future possibilities. The attachment to such negative feelings leads to a predictable continuance of more of the same: bitterness, suppression and suffering in some way.[3]

If you feel that offering forgiveness is impossible, or if you are afraid to face the emotions of past traumas, you are not alone. As hard as it may seem, it is possible to offer forgiveness despite your anger, disappointment or feelings of injustice. Your act of forgiveness will foster an untold amount of courage, which will carry you through any fears you will encounter in the future.

Tanya's Herstory

Among the many interviews I have conducted and people whom I have coached about forgiveness, a woman named Tanya proved to me that no matter how traumatic the circumstance or event, everyone can find the courage to forgive.

Tanya's brother raped her repeatedly as a child. When she finally told her parents about it at the age of seven, they were horrified. In order to keep their son's transgressions from being exposed and to protect him from going to jail, Tanya's parents sent her away from home. They never explained why or even sympathized with their daughter about the situation. They felt that Tanya would be safer in a new environment with no men.

Tanya felt rejected from their home and abandoned by her parents. She thought that they sided with her brother, and she consequently developed a deep distrust for adults. She used fashion and her keen sense of style to seek approval—a classic example of the Beauty Aficionado.

No matter how many compliments she received, it was never enough to quell her fears of rejection. Although she felt violated by her brother, she wanted the intimate attention of men because it was familiar. She valued this familiarity more than neglect. To counter her fear of abandonment, she developed a sweet, submissive disposition and became quite clingy in relationships.

Tanya had never been in a relationship for more than one year. She was losing all hope of having a stable relationship with a man who would not take advantage of her desperate need for intimacy. The voice in her head would not let her forget her past. It told her that she was worthless and that people would always mistreat her.

Tanya was tired of being a victim, so she began an inquiry into what it would take to break through her Herstory. She forgave her mother and father, even though her father had already passed away. Tanya was amazed at the unexpected closeness that occurred in her relationship with her mother; however, shortly after, her mother passed on as well. Tanya felt complete in her relationship with both of her parents, and the weight on her soul seemed to lighten.

Then, after avoiding her brother for 25 years, Tanya found the courage to confront him face to face. Although she dreaded going to the penitentiary where her brother was serving time for repeated acts of violent sexual assault, she wanted to absolve herself from the trauma of her past and move forward with her life. Tanya offered forgiveness and accepted him as her brother. He did not offer Tanya any words of comfort or remorse.

For Tanya, the real rewards lay in being able to face the person—the cause of her appalling memories—and express her pain. She understood that her brother was dealing with deep sociopathic issues and was unable to show compassion for his deeds. The courage Tanya showed by confronting her demons gave her confidence that she never imagined was possible in her life.

Before Tanya forgave her family, she was stuck in a dead-end job doing the minimum to get by. Afterward, Tanya started a new business, which she has operated successfully for over 10 years. Tanya was never able to spend a lot of time on her own because of her fear of abandonment. Now she takes trips by herself to explore, relax and be at peace with her thoughts. She volunteers at a local Boys and Girls Club and loves leading activities to teach the children about healthy communication in relationships. She says that it is her way of "paying it all forward."

Right before she forgave her brother, Tanya began a relationship with a man whom she really cared for. Their relationship immediately blossomed into a connection unlike any relationship she had ever experienced. They have been together for over 11 years! Because of her willingness to confront the person who haunted her, Tanya became the master of her domain and is no longer a victim of her past.

Bring Forgiveness into Your Life

Louise L. Hay is one of my favorite authors. In her book *You Can Heal Your Life,* she discusses the fallout that results from holding on to resentment: "I had had a very difficult childhood with a lot of abuse—mental, physical and sexual. But that was many years ago, and it was no excuse for the way I was treating myself now. I was literally eating my body with cancerous growth because I had not forgiven."[4]

> *When you are willing to restore love to places in your life where you lost sight of it, you can experience the beauty in yourself, in others and in the world.*

I have not found any medical research that proves resentment can cause cancer. However, Hay has been a cancer survivor for decades. I believe she realized that releasing her resentment was instrumental in healing her body.

When you are willing to restore love to places in your life where you lost sight of it, you can experience the beauty in yourself, in others and in the world. Without forgiveness, it is impossible to appreciate your beauty and the essence of who you really are.

Learning to forgive as a way of life replaces your oppressive behavior patterns with positivity. It creates a space in which to build the foundation for feeling beautiful. However, before genuine forgiveness can take root in your heart, you need to clear some debris from the space. It is time to dismantle the origins of your continuing heartbreak and resentment by exposing the negative feelings you hold around your Herstory.

It is normal to feel nervous or even fearful doing these next few exercises. Be gentle with yourself, because self-compassion will make this process much easier. Remember: I let the phone ring 19 times at my parents' house before I talked to my father. Do not give up! You are worth the rewards found on the other side of resentment.

If you are at a place where your Herstory no longer weighs heavily on your heart, then it is time to bring forgiveness to the people in your Herstory. If you have not let go of the significance of your Herstory in order to offer forgiveness, it may be helpful to revisit the "Read Through Your Herstory" exercise in Chapter 4. Once you *have* let go of the emotional charge around your Herstory, you are ready to deliver forgiveness.

Exercise: Forgive and Let Go of Past Hurts

- **Location:** A quiet place where you will not be disturbed

- **Materials:** A few sheets of lined loose-leaf paper, a pencil or pen and a timer

- **Set your timer for:** 30–45 minutes of uninterrupted time, or as long as it takes to write out everything you need to say in order to feel complete with the person to whom you are offering forgiveness

- **Preparation:** Take five minutes to go within and quiet your mind.

- **Instructions:** Start by writing a letter that offers forgiveness to and asks forgiveness from the person/people in your Herstory. You can email your letter or send it through the mail, but I highly recommend reading it to the person over the phone or in person, if possible.

Follow these criteria for writing your letter:

- Use "I" whenever possible. This places the responsibility for the situation on you and avoids shifting any blame to the recipient of the letter. Taking responsibility for what happened gives you power.

- Use past tense to show that you are really giving up that blame. Let them know exactly what actions you blamed them for, such as:

  ° "I blamed you for not showing me how to love."

  ° "I blamed you for making me feel inferior."

  ° "I blamed you for me growing up too fast. I've realized that blaming you keeps me _____."
  (Fill in the impact of your blame. This could mean revealing that you were stuck in predictable patterns or filled with negative emotions such as feeling distant and unfulfilled.)

- Then, use the present tense to show that you are done blaming them:

  ° "I am now ready to stop putting the burden on you and take responsibility for my feelings. I forgive you."

- Here are the next steps:

  ° "Will you forgive me for blaming you for _____?"
  (Fill in whatever you wrote above.)

○ "I am ready to take responsibility for my life and put this behind us. The way I would like us to relate to each other from now on is _____." (Fill in the kind of relationship you would like to have with this person, and make a promise concerning how you will treat them going forward.)

Exercise: Release Others Whom You Have Condemned

- **Location:** A place where you can have a private conversation or think clearly to write this letter

- **Materials:** A telephone, Internet and email access, and a timer

- **Set your timer for:** 60–90 minutes of uninterrupted time

- **Preparation:** Take five minutes to go within and quiet your mind.

- **Instructions:** Before you make that phone call or send that letter, see if it passes the criteria outlined in the last exercise by asking a trusted friend to read it. Ask them to tell you if they hear even a *hint* of righteousness, blame or resentment.

After your friend approves your letter, you are ready to contact the other person. If the person whom you are forgiving is no longer alive, ask your trusted friend to play the role of that person. Read the letter to them.

Once you have read your letter, thank them for allowing you to express yourself. The other party is not always going to receive you or your heartfelt attempt at forgiveness positively. Prepare for the worst and expect the best.

With an open heart, hear whatever they may need to say. They have made up their own interpretation of the past and may or may not be experiencing a negative impact from it. Show them compassion. The best thing you can do is to listen to them. Resist the urge to justify or defend yourself, and thank them for sharing.

Practicing daily forgiveness is a great way to keep your mindset positive. At the end of each day, right before I go to sleep, I say a small prayer asking for forgiveness from anyone who may have felt that I did something wrong to them.

I also offer forgiveness to anyone I may have cast out of my heart, cut off communication with, passed harsh judgments on, gossiped about, or blamed for any failures or hardships I have experienced.

I write out what happened with that person, and I read it many times. I read the past event until I separate the meaning I attached to the situation from the events that actually transpired. I try to make amends immediately. Even if it is something small, such as someone not excusing himself or herself for stepping on my toe while riding the subway, I direct my forgiveness to that person.

The more letters and conversations you have with people you regard with contempt, the easier forgiveness will become. The easier forgiveness becomes, the more compassion you will have for yourself and others.

While makeup can cover surface imperfections, forgiveness can completely make over and restore your spirit.

CHAPTER 6

Beauty's True Source—
How to Trust and Listen
to Your Higher Self

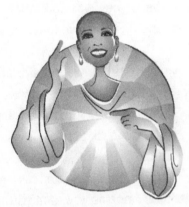

Give me beauty in the inward soul;
and may the inner and the outer be at one.

—Socrates

On My Own

After eleven years of friendship and seven years of marriage with my husband, I found myself in a tiny studio apartment in Los Angeles—alone. It was different from the lifestyle to which I was accustomed, but it was a starting point to reinvent "me."

I had previously connected my identity to being someone's wife. Aside from living on a college campus, this was the first time in my adult life that I was on my own. Even in college, I never *really* felt completely on my own.

Although I felt liberated, I was left with a big void in my life. After separating from my husband and letting go of the resentment I had toward my father, I felt as if I were starting over from nothing. I didn't know who I was or what I wanted for myself. I was approaching 30, and this was not at all what I imagined my life would look like at this age. Many of my friends back in Chicago were well into their careers, married and having their first or second baby. I had none of that.

I spent many nights crying myself to sleep and even more waking hours in deep contemplation. At times, I was certain that I had made the right decision; at other times, the fact that I had deliberately turned my life inside out and upside down bewildered me.

Was I stupid?

I was going through what I suppose were the normal stages of grieving the loss of a loved one, and it was not easy. Every day, I managed to wake up and go to work. However, there were times when I would rush into a bathroom, or to the back storage area at work, to cry my eyes out. Everyone around me was new, so I didn't feel as though I had much of a support group to comfort me and reassure me that I would be all right. It was definitely not easy, but after a few months, my emotions stabilized. I felt ready to move forward . . . but *how?*

Though I needed to find the "me" that was somehow lost in the relationship I had with my husband, I focused on my exterior instead of my spiritual and emotional well-being. I changed everything about my looks, from eyebrows to toenails, in an effort to revitalize myself.

> *After a short time, I made up my mind that if I couldn't have the fairy-tale life, I would at least **look** like I did.*

During that time, it seemed logical to work on my physical appearance. It was easier than dealing with the social stigma of being single and living alone. Instead of relying on my intuition to guide me through this period of change, I looked to the world around me to figure out how I should look and feel at this stage in my life.

After a short time, I made up my mind that if I couldn't have the fairy-tale life, I would at least *look* like I did.

Then, my teacher arrived.

As the saying goes, "When the student is ready, the teacher will appear." And appear she did!

My Neighbor's Style and Allure

My next-door neighbor was a beautiful, lighthearted, extremely feminine and appearance-conscious Lebanese woman—a true Beauty Authority. Every detail about her appearance was always intact. In the months that I observed her, I never saw her leave her apartment looking like a mess.

She had a great sense of style, and she seemed to know exactly the right thing to wear for every occasion. She possessed an allure to which men seemed to flock—almost as if she had a spell over them. In my observation of her, I was trying to find out if I needed what she had. The perfect storm was brewing within me, and I was falling into the second classic beauty block. I was making harsh comparisons that were unfair to me.

This exploration did not stop with my neighbor. Month in and month out, I looked through countless magazines—including *Elle, Vogue, Essence, InStyle* and *Women's Fitness,* to name a few—trying to find the "me" that I thought I had lost. But the "me" I was looking for never seemed to appear. I began to think that I wasn't capable of finding myself on my own, a thought process that drew me into a whirlwind of constant comparison of myself to other women I thought had characteristics I needed or wanted more of.

I thought that in order to make my outward appearance reflect my new life, I would need help from the beauty authorities who had it all together. I befriended my neighbor and, instead of learning from our friendship that she was just as quirky and beautifully human as the next girl, I continued to compare the features about her that I admired most with parts of myself that I found lacking.

Though I don't think I ever expressed it to her, my neighbor became my style guru and my support. While hanging out at her place one day, she noticed that I was tugging at my clothing—something I often did. Being a very forward person that often said exactly what was on her mind—a quality I quite admired in her—she quickly put me in my place.

"Where have you been living?" she asked sharply. "A hole in Baghdad?"

I could tell by her smile that she was joking but also making a point. She took me by the hand and pulled me toward her full-length mirror. As she tugged at my clothes and held my face at different angles, gently forcing me to look at myself, I anticipated the worse.

"You are so beautiful, and you are hiding it all! What is it that you don't want people to see? You've got a great body, a beautiful face and an amazing personality!"

I smiled at her. For the first time, I could actually hear her words as *the truth*.

"Why do you dress like this, Kenetia? No one can see the real you!"

She walked out of the room and left me staring at my reflection. Even though I was laughing aloud with her, on the inside I felt as if she had struck a sensitive nerve.

Where was I hiding the real "me"?

Reinventing Myself and Falling from Grace

For the next several months, I spent a ton of time and more money than I actually had trying to find myself. I felt moments of happiness and fulfillment while buying sexy, sassy clothes I would have previously looked down my nose at. Instead of hiding behind my clothes and ignoring my appearance, I was doing the exact opposite. My look had undeniably improved. My new wardrobe was a bit more revealing, and the attention I desired was coming my way. I wasn't necessarily feeling more like *me* though.

In the meantime, I became less than enthusiastic about my job and started to feel completely trapped. I did not see a way to advance my career as a freelance makeup artist without the support of my husband or a full-time job. My credit card bills were piling up, and my anxiety level was rising right along with them.

It was the holiday season. I was broke, lonely and feeling completely hopeless about the mounting debt that I incurred during my fruitless obsession to find myself. No matter how much I tried to avoid dealing with my emotions by improving my appearance, it never seemed to work for any length of time. Immediately after I bought a few nice things, such as makeup or clothes, I would feel very good about myself. I would wear the clothes a couple of times, and then the thrill would disappear. Inevitably, I quickly returned to that frustrating feeling of not measuring up.

The clock struck midnight—a new year with nothing to celebrate. I was home alone watching television, when my body broke down from a sudden, excruciating abdominal pain unlike any pain I had ever felt.

I drove myself to the hospital. After 10 hours in the emergency room and two doctors telling me that they could not find anything wrong, they sent me home with an antacid and a $10,000 medical bill.

At home, the pain in my stomach subsided a bit, but I still felt physically weak and emotionally drained. I wanted so badly to curl up in a ball and cry, but the silence in my room was so profound that I did not want to interfere with it.

Three hours later, I managed to pull myself together and go to work. Although I wasn't happy with my job, I certainly was not prepared to leave it. My life was in complete disarray, and I felt to my core that I had fallen from grace.

My mind continued to ask the same questions I had asked myself before:

"Why did my life look like this?"

"Why am I here all alone?"

"Why do I hate my job?"

"Where is that light, vibrant, beautiful person other people say I am?"

"*Why am I here?*"

Four hours after that, I was in bed again, staring at the same spot on the ceiling. *They fired me!*

> I was learning an important life lesson—that the momentary satisfaction of a new exterior enhancement is never enough to fill a lingering void in the soul.

In one breath, I was devastated; in the next breath, I was completely relieved.

"Now what?"

Every possible emotion ran through me, and I started to weep. I was newly separated from my husband, had no job and very little savings. My family was back in Chicago, and I could see no options for myself, none at all.

Every area of my life looked like (excuse my French) *shit!* I could barely stand to look at myself in the mirror. Even with my new-and-improved body, clothes and makeup, my self-esteem was at an all-time low. I was learning an important life lesson—that the momentary satisfaction of a new exterior enhancement is never enough to fill a lingering void in the soul.

The Downside of Smoke and Mirrors

Instead of cultivating an understanding of who I was, I opted instead for a false representation. My life was a mess, and I wanted to make it appear as if it were a bed of roses. I was not being honest with myself about the impact of my separation and the choices I made. I turned to the world around me as a distraction from all of the painful regrets for which I condemned myself.

Instead of taking the time to experience the upsetting feelings or ensuing changes in our lives, women are more likely to fuss, obsess or feel oppressed about their appearance. This is a primary way we can hide, ignore or avoid coping with pressing issues.

This may sound like a general statement. But I hear it over and over again from women throughout the country who have gone through major life change, such as divorce, the loss of a job or the loss of a firm belly after pregnancy. They do the same thing I did: seek advice from magazines, celebrities, plastic surgeons and next-door neighbors in an attempt to mend themselves.

In most cases, these actions leave the individual emotionally, physically and, oftentimes, financially bankrupt, bringing her full circle, right back to the emotions she was trying to avoid.

The emotions I desperately wanted to avoid were guilt, shame and disappointment. In many ways, I felt like a failure in marriage, money matters and health. I wept for hours on my bed, as if I were purging all of my unfulfilled expectations. I cried as if doing so could release me from all of the wrong I thought I had created.

Amidst the tears of my completely weakened and vulnerable state, I heard a tiny voice from within gently whisper: *trust yourself.*

Trust myself?

The very thought of trusting myself made me angry. Chills ran over my body. I questioned why this message would be relevant now.

I wondered, "Why should I *trust* myself when all I've done is make a big *mess* of things? What do *I* know? I wouldn't be in this place if I could *trust* myself!"

Then, something occurred to me. Throughout my life, I was the one person that no one ever taught me to trust. Growing up, I learned to trust my parents and the adults they entrusted me with, including my teachers, relatives and their friends. Being raised a Christian, the church taught me to place my trust in God and the folks reading from the Bible in front of the church. Throughout my schooling, I learned to trust textbooks but never myself.

Why now?

Taking a Leap of Faith

After hours of screaming and weeping, I lay on my side and stared at the books on my bookshelf. I spotted *The Seven Spiritual Laws of Success* by Deepak Chopra—a medical doctor, author and speaker on spirituality who helps people understand the ways in which the mind, body and spirit work together.

I picked up the book and turned to the very last page. I read the information included about the Chopra Center, which was near San Diego. I had read the book on and off over the course of 10 years and often thought that if I were ever in California, I would go to this center and meet Dr. Chopra himself.

Once I was able to catch my breath, I called the Chopra Center and signed up for a four-day wellness retreat. I had just enough money to float me through the next couple of months' rent and to pay for this retreat. Although it felt illogical to spend this amount of money on something unproven, I took a leap of faith.

The following Wednesday, I found myself driving my car from Los Angeles to San Diego. I checked into my hotel room, dropped my bags on the floor and walked straight to the mirror. I was not pleased at my overall reflection: I looked haggard. My skin was dull. My eyes were tired. And beneath all of that, I felt sad, angry, frustrated and worthless.

> *I felt a renewed sense of peace, harmony and confidence, qualities I had been missing for years.*

At the Chopra Center, I sat among a group of six strangers and felt emotionally exhausted, mentally frustrated and physically worn out. I craved a miracle to fix my mess.

When I looked in the mirror five days later, *I could see and feel my magnificence* for the first time. I was floating on air. I felt vibrant and full of life. I felt a renewed sense of peace, harmony and confidence, qualities I had been missing for years. My mind, body and spirit were finally in alignment.

I had acquired solid, daily practices to keep me grounded in my newly found awareness. I had learned how to manage my entire well-being through food, body movement, bodywork, yoga, journaling and meditation. I was full of energy, yet I was enjoying a profound sense of peace. I was ready to face the world.

Even though my daily practices didn't provide answers as to how I was going to get myself out of the crazy mess that I had created, I was no longer worried about it. Every day, I kept true to my practice of meditation, well-balanced meals, body movement and journaling.

When I looked at myself in the mirror, it was as if I had undergone a facelift—but better—because my eyes recognized my beauty. In my heart, I actually felt *beautiful*. Having experienced my own beauty for the first time in years, I remembered why I started my career as a makeup artist in the first place: to understand what really made a woman feel beautiful. This inquiry became my mission.

The Start of a Successful Career

Weeks later, none of my circumstances had changed, but I stayed true to my practice and newly found mission. With this in mind, I attended a workshop to improve my makeup skills. During the workshop, I met a young woman who excitedly shared that she had just come from an interview with Revlon and was about to embark on a 25-city tour promoting their newest mascara.

Without much thought, I asked, "Do you know if they are still hiring?"

"I believe their last day of interviewing was yesterday, but here is the lady's number."

The next morning, I called the agency that was hiring on Revlon's behalf.

"Hello. My name is Kenetia. I heard that you were looking for makeup artists from Los Angeles to tour the country. I also heard that your interview process was completed a couple of days ago; however, I wanted to know if you would consider adding me to your roster of potential candidates."

"Sure!" she said. "Email me a picture, resume and bio. I'll pass it along to the selection committee."

Within minutes, I emailed her my information. I was so excited that

I forgot to ask about the logistics of the tour, such as how long it would last, how much I would earn or when I might hear back from her. As soon as I sent the email, I let it go. I kept up my search to find work as a freelance makeup artist and continued to set up photo shoots to build my portfolio.

The following Tuesday morning, I sat in my studio and meditated. During the middle of my meditation, a soft, quiet voice suggested that I open my eyes. The second I did, I saw my phone flashing and displaying a New York area code. The voice on the other end was filled with excitement.

"Kenetia, we would like you to join us as one of the elite team of eight makeup artists to travel with us to the top 25 markets promoting Revlon's new mascara. We need you to fly to New York City this Sunday to start training on Monday."

"*Yes*, I'd love to!"

Within five days, I packed my entire studio and arranged for someone to live there and pay my rent for the three months that I would be touring the country. This exciting new start to a successful career as a makeup artist was the physical evidence I needed to know that it was safe to trust my intuition.

Your Intuitive Voice

If it were not for my complete meltdown in my tiny studio apartment, I am not sure I would have heard that little voice telling me to trust myself. Awakenings come to us at various points in life, and not always because of a complete breakdown. It is possible to recognize when you need to embrace forgiveness and trust yourself without having your entire life implode. However, when your life *does* implode, you become present to all of the choices you made that went completely against your intuition.

When I doubt myself or rely more on others for direction, it is a clear sign that I do not trust myself to make the right decision. Doubting my skill as a makeup artist prevented me hundreds of times from calling photographers and production companies. When I asked my maid of honor the night before my wedding if she thought that I could learn to love my future husband, it was another instance of me not listening to my intuition.

Every time I do not trust my ability to make my own choices, I create more problems for myself. Ignoring my intuition leaves me questioning my actions. I talk about what I *should* do instead of doing what I know needs to be done. My energy gets very low, and I find it challenging to focus. It is natural to inquire of yourself and others in order to achieve clarity and think things through. However, when your intellect overpowers your gut instincts, it is a sure sign that it is time to go within and listen for what you *truly* want.

By adopting a daily practice of meditation, your desires become clear, and you learn to trust your "intuitive voice" with ease. This voice is distinctly different from that of your Delusional Diva.

Your intuition serves to guide you toward your truest expression; your Delusional Diva serves to protect you from the illusion of fear. Following your intuition can be a bit scary because the Diva's logical thought patterns can seem saner—or safer—than your intuitive ways of thinking.

You may intuitively know that if you head in a particular direction, it will result in your happiness. However, because you are not sure about the steps you need to take, or exactly what will happen on that journey, you may become fearful. This is when your Delusional Diva kicks in to protect you from uncertainty. Because of that fear, you choose the safer, more rational—but not necessarily better—option.

My intuitive voice spoke to me that I should sign up for a workshop after recently losing my job. The same voice told me to speak up and get the phone number for a job for which someone else had already applied. My rational thinking voice—the one with all the reasons and concerns—would have backed away from both opportunities out of fear of uncertainty or fear of stepping on someone else's toes.

Listening to Your Intuition Takes Courage

Because your intuitive voice defies your Delusional Diva's protective nature, it takes courage to believe that your intuitive voice has your best interest at heart. Your intuition has no fear filters. It is motivated solely by what you really want from life.

Below are a few questions that I have learned to ask myself when faced with making decisions at a moment's notice. These questions help me determine if my intuitive voice is speaking to me or if my Delusional Diva is running the show:

- "Will this bring me happiness?"

- "Am I doing this just to get by?"

- "Does this feel right, or is this just the easy or popular option?"

- "Is the reward greater than the risk, or am I just afraid to fail?"

- "Will I regret this?"

If you avoid asking yourself questions that begin with "What if," you have a greater chance of steering clear of your Delusional Diva's protective reasoning. Life starts to happen when you move past your fears and start trusting your intuition. When you accept that your intuition has your best interest at heart and that it does not want to lead you down a path of unhappiness or suffering, you will start to follow your intuition consistently.

Deepen Your Connection to Your Intuitive Voice

You may not always know where you are going when you listen to your intuition, but you will always know that you are living your life the way you want to live it—instead of just *getting through* your life. The following are a few guided meditations to facilitate building a deeper, stronger connection with your intuitive voice.

Exercise: Meditation to Build Self-Trust

- **Location:** A quiet place where you will not be disturbed

- **Materials:** Pen or pencil, journal or paper, and a timer

- **Set your timer for:** 30 minutes of uninterrupted time

- **Preparation:** Take five minutes to go within and quiet your mind.

- **Instructions:** Unlike the previous exercises in this book, the results of this exercise are going to happen over time. If you have a hard time trusting yourself, you are not alone. If you haven't started to meditate and you are interested in receiving the benefits of trusting yourself, now is the perfect time to begin.

Before going into your silent meditation, I want you to spend a maximum of two minutes contemplating and answering these universal questions:

- "Who am I?"

- "What do I really want?"

- "What is my purpose in life?"

When I am searching for an answer to a situation that I am second-guessing, I change the second question ("What do I really want?") to:

- "What is my desired outcome from this situation?"

- "What would be for the highest good?"

Immediately after meditating, take a few minutes to journal about any insights that have come to you. Write out the first two or three fears that come to mind about the choice you are contemplating.

Making journal entries like these will help you identify if you have acted from that still, quiet voice or from your fears. When you witness that your still, quiet voice consistently produces your desired outcomes, you will learn that trusting yourself is, by far, your best bet.

Exercise: Meditation for Self-Forgiveness

- **Location:** A quiet place where you will not be disturbed

- **Materials:** Pen or pencil, journal or paper, and a timer

- **Set your timer for:** 30 minutes of uninterrupted time, including five to ten minutes to journal

- **Preparation:** Take five minutes to go within and quiet your mind.

- **Instructions:** If forgiving yourself is challenging, or if you have lingering regrets about the choices you have made in your life, use this meditation to let go of those negative emotions about yourself. This meditation will help you develop compassion and wash away any unfulfilled expectations that you have for yourself.

Before going into your silent meditation, spend a maximum of two minutes contemplating the following statements:

- "I am whole, perfect and complete."

- "I always do the best I can in any given situation."

- "My experiences are a function of me learning more about myself."

Immediately after meditating, take a few minutes to journal about any insights that have come to you. When you do this exercise over a period of three weeks, it will help you break free from any guilt, blame or shame that you have placed on yourself.

After three weeks of doing this exercise three or four times a week, read your journal entries and take note of any consistent themes. Be patient with yourself and the forgiveness will flow to you.

When I learned to quiet my Delusional Diva's doubt, worry and fear through meditation and began asking thoughtful questions to guide me to my highest good, I found that I could trust myself more than I could trust anyone else. I learned to make decisions for myself that created the experiences that I most desired.

Learning to connect with your divine intelligence within is one of the greatest gifts you can ever give yourself. Trusting your *intuition* makes life simpler and, in many cases, magical. There is no longer any reason to look to the world around you to find out if you measure up or to determine if you are making the right life decisions.

Best of all, trusting yourself allows you to govern your life and create the beauty you want to experience from a place of authenticity and inspiration.

CHAPTER 7

Actualizing Beauty—
Reclaiming the Fearless Child
within You

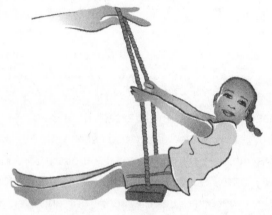

In search of my mother's garden, I found my own.
—Alice Walker

"Mirror, Mirror, on the Wall . . ."

Before the incident at Rachel's house, I would spend hours playing in front of the mirror. I dressed up in different clothes, pretended to be cartoon characters and imitated others' facial expressions. There was complete acceptance of the miniature person staring back at me—judgment and criticism had not yet entered the picture. My fascination was one of pure curiosity and wonder of just *being*.

As I grew older, and as my Herstory unfolded, the positive feelings that had accompanied my playtimes in front of the mirror gave way to feelings of dread. Maybe it was my observations of the adults around me who showed disdain for their reflection, or maybe it was my entrance into grade school where kids made it painfully clear that my forehead was something from a creature feature. Whatever the reasons, the mirror began to represent a place for self-criticism. Despite years of my parents and relatives affirming how beautiful I was, once I started school, those affirmations vanished.

Every time I looked in the mirror, all I could see was my forehead. My schoolmates gave it nasty little nicknames, such as "snow globe," "crystal ball" and "egghead"—all meaning that it was larger than a normal forehead.

As I moved out of elementary school into junior high and then high school, my attention shifted away from my forehead to the rest of my body's imperfections. I had thick hips, thick thighs and big boobs— every teenage girl's wish, I guess, except for mine.

I picked apart every inch of my body each time I walked in front of a mirror. I was in a constant self-battle about my round butt, square hips, chubby arms, skinny legs . . . (The list went on forever.) The remarks from others were insulting, upsetting and even demeaning, but they were nothing like the cruel banter I shared with myself about my perceived flaws.

Gone were the days when my time in front of the mirror represented total acceptance and freedom.

Remember the Evil Queen who demanded praise in *Snow White?* Let us revisit that fairy-tale princess story and recall when she looked into the mirror to ask the famous question:

"Mirror, mirror, on the wall. Who's the fairest of them all?"

Naturally, the mirror replied, "You are, My Lady."

If your mirror had the ability to grant such high praise, would you kindly accept the compliment or would you argue relentlessly to convince the mirror of how wrong it was, no matter what it told you?

During my career, I have been "the mirror" for hundreds of women— Victoria's Secret models, Miss Universe contestants, Wall Street stock brokers and moms—and I can attest that women are far more likely to wage war against praise they feel is inaccurate or undeserved than to embrace it. If mirrors were able to play back to you on a loud-speaker the intense self-criticism that lies within you as you look at your reflection, you would feel justified in breaking them!

Instead of breaking mirrors, I think it is time to break the unusually cruel relationship that women develop between themselves and the mirror. It is time to reclaim that fearless, playful, childlike wonder again! Self-criticism is largely a learned behavior that women adopt from observing other women. The mirror does not have to be a place for criticism and judgment. It is possible to make friends with the reflection you see every day and return to a place of acceptance and appreciation of the person standing before you.

It is possible to make friends with the reflection you see every day and return to a place of acceptance and appreciation of the person standing before you.

When you fill your heart with forgiveness and compassion, your conversation about your reflection softens. Your thoughts about your physical reflection reconnect with that bright, joyful child who simply got lost with time.

Stop Making Unfair Comparisons

You can break your mirror-bashing banter by refraining from unfair comparisons. These comparisons concerning your physical beauty, relationships, financial status or career do not give you an opportunity to blaze your own pathway, especially when they determine where you *should* be in life or how you *should* look.

Making comparisons in this way is a setup for absolute failure, namely when you use them to gauge whether or not you measure up. Remember, there is no one on this planet like you, and there never will be. So who on earth should you look like besides you?

Here are some common statements you may say to yourself that create comparisons that work against you:

- "I'm too fat." (Compared to whom?)

- "I should look like her." (Are your genes and her genes an identical match?)

- "These jeans used to fit." (When did they fit? Six years ago?)

- "My nose is too big." (Whose nose, other than yours, are you looking at?)

- "I should be a size 8." (Says who? The last time I checked, there are many sizes in department stores.)

- "My cheeks look like balloons." (Do they look like hot-air balloons or helium party balloons?)

OK, I'm having some fun with this, but you get the idea. If you become present to what you are actually saying, including recognizing to what or to whom you are comparing yourself, you will gain a sense of self-compassion instead of constant criticism.

Pure observation without judgment will help you learn what you like and don't like. Comparing your observations to how you should or shouldn't look, or where you should or shouldn't be in your life, is a recipe for unhappiness and unrest.

> It is your responsibility to make the choices that will bring your actual life into closer alignment with your unique vision for your life.

Using comparisons in a productive way can help you develop a better understanding of your wants and desires. The trick is to limit your comparisons to personal experiences. Do not compare yourself to others as I did with my neighbor. Do not even compare your old self with who you are now. Only make comparisons in the context of whether or not what you experienced is something you want to experience again.

It is your responsibility to make the choices that will bring your actual life into closer alignment with your unique vision for your life.

If you make judgments about the way things should or should not be, rather than being with the way they are, you will not be creating from a place of inspiration. Instead, you will be creating out of fear, worry and lack. This will keep you unsatisfied.

Focus on What You Love

Another way to transform your critical self-commentary in the mirror is to look for what you love about yourself. My mantra is, "Find what you love and forgive the rest."

Below are some suggestions that will help you reclaim the beauty in your reflection:

- Don't spend countless hours in front of the mirror worrying about your imperfections.

- Don't journal about all the reasons you hate your nose.

- Don't call up your friends and spend hours talking about how much you don't like your body's imperfections.

- Don't hang out in groups that gossip about their ugliness.

- Find something about your physical appearance that you already like.

- Find ways to focus your attention on the attributes you like about yourself. Whenever your eyes and wandering mind go down that dark tunnel, readjust your attention to those things you love.

When you focus on what you love, what you do not like will take a backseat by default. This is called "mind over matter." I'll be the first to admit that this isn't always an easy concept to apply when it comes to the physical body—especially if you experience your body acting in a way that is abnormal to you. For example, when you get a pimple on your face, all you see when you look in the mirror is that pimple, right? Then, all of a sudden, it gets bigger or others pop up all around it.

When we focus our thoughts on the problem, in this case the pimple, we tend to experience more of the problem. This does not happen just by chance. Your attention and thoughts are very powerful magnets that attract what you think about most. The more energy and attention you give something, the faster you will attract it.

By focusing such energy and attention on your pimples, you increase the likelihood of more pimples. Conversely, if you focus on clear, healthy skin, you will inevitably attract, seek out and find ways to have healthy, clear skin.

I believe that you will be able to see and feel your beauty more clearly when you focus your attention on those parts of yourself you most love and feel are desirable. Jennifer Nardozzi, PsyD, a clinical psychologist specializing in the treatment of women with eating disorders and the National Training Manager at the Renfrew Center in Miami, had much to say about this topic in a recent interview:

This will probably sound very lame, but we can't change certain things. We can't change our parents. We can't change some of the childhood experiences we've had. We can't change some of our failures. We can't change our genetics. You can't change that you are going to be 5'6" if you are only going to be 5'5". There are things that you absolutely can't change, but there are things that you can change, in terms of your attitude toward what occurred in your life or in terms of what you are going to create here on Earth.

The more we can just accept that things have happened, we experience more peace. When you stop focusing on all the things that have gone wrong or all the things that are wrong with your body, and instead focus on the things that are right about you, you experience more peace.

How did those really, really hard things that happened in your life make you who you are? How did those things give you strength and courage? So many things are right with you. So, you don't particularly love your hips. It is okay. What is it that you *do* love about you? Where are you going to turn your attention?

I think that each of us has a choice, in terms of what we are going to choose to focus on. If you focus on the negative, you produce negativity. If you focus on the positive, you produce the positive.[1]

Courtney's Herstory

A few years ago, I coached a woman named Courtney who desperately wanted to improve her self-image. Courtney became significantly overweight at a very young age. Her mother always told her that if she ever wanted to find a nice guy who wanted to be with her, she would have to lose weight.

She grew up believing that people who have good relationships with men must be thin. Naturally, when she became an adult, she had a hard time finding a mate because she thought that only thin women had good relationships. Men treated her coldly and showed her little interest.

She really wanted a relationship, so she committed to losing weight—a *lot* of weight. After putting a thinner version of herself into the dating world, she came to the conclusion that what her mom told her was untrue.

Courtney found that men were just as unkind to her when she was thin as when she was heavy. She continued to be alone while watching her heavy and thin friends find joy in their relationships, whether dating or engaged. She realized that there was something deeper, beyond her weight and figure, that required attention. That's when she contacted me.

Once we unraveled Courtney's Herstory, she discovered that she had interpreted her mother's statement to mean that she would never be good enough for a man. Because she thought that people would see what a scared, worthless, unattractive person she was, Courtney became fearful about being in social situations. She was extremely introverted and lived in a shell. She would talk very little about herself and was "boring on dates" (her words, not mine).

Courtney came to grips with her Herstory. She understood that her mom *thought* she was doing the right thing by telling her daughter that she would not meet a nice man unless she was thin. Through a few conversations with her mom, she learned that her mother's comments, although hurtful, were out of love. They were merely beliefs that her mother had learned during her upbringing. As is the case with most parents, she was just doing what she thought was best for her daughter.

Courtney eventually forgave her mom. More importantly, Courtney asked her mom for forgiveness for blaming her for a self-inflicted situation. She also learned to stop making comparisons with others through an exercise I taught her over the course of a few weeks.

This exercise, which I have shared at the end of this chapter, taught her to listen to and observe those moments when she made comparisons that diminished her self-esteem. She learned to identify these moments that prevented her from trusting in her divine design.

Courtney has gained weight back; however, this time, she has learned to appreciate her curves as her body's genuine expression. When she initially lost so much weight, it was partly due to comparing herself with other women instead of gauging what felt good and comfortable for *her*. She actually felt uncomfortable and even more self-conscious being "skinny" than she felt when she was "pleasantly plump."

Now, she eats what she wants without drowning herself in food. She maintains a comfortable, healthy weight and loves the way she looks— so do the men she dates! She no longer looks to men for validation or shakes in fear of their judgments. She enjoys the process of dating. Men compliment her figure and the dimples in her legs because she is confident in her femininity which, to her, is sexy. She feels soft, lovable and worthy of love.

Courtney is more outgoing because of the way she feels, yet she still finds inspiration in her introversion. She discovered that she had hidden talents. She couldn't begin to explore these talents when she was constantly comparing herself with others. As soon as she looked within herself, however, she found the experiences she truly wanted. Now, she embraces her newfound abilities to sing, write and paint. She regularly shows her paintings in galleries and sings at open mic nights.

Exercise: Make Comparisons Without Condemning Yourself

- **Location:** A quiet place where you will not be disturbed

- **Materials:** A journal, pen and paper, mental awareness throughout your day, and a timer

- **Set your timer for:** 60–90 minutes of uninterrupted time

- **Preparation:** Take five minutes to go within and quiet your mind.

- **Instructions:** The purpose of this exercise is to help you stop making comparisons that diminish your worth. It will help you appreciate who you are, where you are from and what you look like. It will also build trust in your process. For this exercise, you will need to make a conscious, daily effort to observe and journal your observations.

It is important to recognize when you are comparing yourself to others. At the beginning of your day, set the intention to observe all of your thoughts. Whenever you find yourself looking at someone and envying something she has, make a mental note.

Take a deep breath and, as you release your breath, release all of the thoughts that flooded your brain and caused a comparison.

In your next breath, focus your thoughts and energy on a part of you that brings you joy. It could be your hair, nails, smile or something you have recently accomplished—direct your attention to what you appreciate about *you*. The more you focus on what is good about you and your life, the less you will feel the urge to make comparisons.

At the end of each day, pull out your journal and answer these questions right before you go to bed:

- How many times did you make comparisons today?

- When you caught yourself making a comparison, what did you focus on to divert your attention back to yourself?

- What is missing about yourself that you want to feel or experience?

- If you discovered that you already possessed what you felt was missing, in what way would you act differently?

At the end of three weeks, go back through your journal and write about the experience of observing yourself while making comparisons.

- Did you decrease or increase the number of times you made comparisons?

- Do you see any consistent patterns or times when you feel triggers to compare yourself to others?

- What, if anything, do you see missing?

- Did you discover anything you would do differently? Did this help boost your confidence in your own abilities

The sooner you are able to catch yourself in the act of making comparisons and divert your attention to those areas of yourself that make you happy, the sooner the time you spend in the mirror will prove to be a fun and playful experience again.

CHAPTER 8

A Declaration of Beauty— Define and Create What Matters Most to You

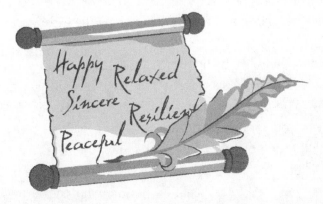

People often say that this or that person has not yet found himself. But the self is not something one finds, it is something one creates.

—Thomas Szasz

Defining Beauty

The definition of beauty is truly personal. I think it is a good idea, however, to read *The Merriam-Webster Dictionary* to help you formulate your definition. Remember, you started to build your definition in Chapter 1's exercise "Ask Yourself about Beauty" on page 23.

> beauty (*n.*)
> **1:** the quality or aggregate of qualities in a person or thing that gives pleasure to the senses or pleasurably exalts the mind or spirit : loveliness
> **2:** a beautiful person or thing; *especially* : a beautiful woman
> **3:** a particularly graceful, ornamental, or excellent quality

Here are a few details I find particularly interesting about these definitions:

- They note *qualities* (not features).

- They point to qualities that are *in* (not *on*) a person or a thing.

- The experience of beauty is one of pleasure to the *senses,* meaning that it is more than just a sense of sight. Beauty exalts the mind or spirit pleasurably, and you feel uplifted by the experience.

Beauty clearly lies within and is comprised of all the qualities you deem pleasing to your senses. Once you know which qualities are pleasing to you, you can start to cultivate those qualities from within.

I invite you to identify qualities that you feel are pleasing. First, I suggest thinking of other people—I know how hard it is to see your own qualities. The point is to identify what you most like and desire.

- When you think of a beautiful person, who comes to mind (e.g., Beyoncé Knowles, Princess Diana, Jennifer Lopez, Elizabeth Taylor, Mahatma Gandhi, Martin Luther King, Jr., Maya Angelou, Brad Pitt, Angelina Jolie, Halle Berry, Oprah Winfrey, Lucy Liu, your neighbor, your mother, your aunt or your uncle)?

- What qualities do you see in them that lead you to think of them as beautiful (e.g., bright, bubbly, charismatic, fun, genuine, energetic or warm)? I am *not* asking you to identify their features (e.g., nose, hair or skin).

List of Pleasing Qualities

Here is a list of pleasing qualities to help you expand your scope:

Physical (body)

healthy	radiant	flexible	gracious
relaxed	toned	strong	

Attitude (mind)

calm	playful	sincere	focused
open	bold	clear	

Emotional (spirit)

vibrant	joyful	excited	forgiving
peaceful	resilient	even	

From this list of pleasing qualities, which ones speak to you?

Your Subconscious Thoughts

Now that you know which qualities of beauty speak to you, making a declaration is easy. A "declaration" is an explicit, formal announcement, either spoken or written, which affirms to you and others how things are in the present tense. It is a clear intention that calls you to act, feel and be a certain way.

Whatever you focus your attention on, you will attract. I believe this is especially true when strong feelings undergird your desires and you put those desires into words. We create our reality through spoken and written words. If you doubt this philosophy, consider how others' words about the way you look or who you are become ingrained in your subconscious. These words may become so real that you forget they *aren't* real. Putting your desires into words is a way to recalibrate your subconscious thoughts so they are building you up instead of tearing you down.

Choose one quality that you find attractive from each of the categories above. These should be qualities you want to become aspects of who you are. Write them here:

_____

_____

_____

In the following exercise, use these words to create a Declaration of Beauty for how you want to experience your unique beauty (body, mind and spirit). These qualities are probably those that you feel are missing when you look in the mirror and cause you to feel dissatisfied about your reflection.

When my mind starts racing because I am focusing energy on what is not right with what I see in the mirror, I pull out my Declaration of Beauty and say it a few times to myself. Before I know it, I have grounded myself once again in what I *want* to feel about myself—not in what is wrong with me.

If you are ready to experience yourself as "beautiful," I will show you how to put together your Declaration of Beauty in this exercise.

Exercise: Create Your Declaration of Beauty

- **Location:** A quiet place where you will not be disturbed and where you feel inspired to create

- **Materials:** Three qualities that most inspire you, a pen or pencil, journal or paper, and a timer

- **Set your timer for:** 10–15 minutes of uninterrupted time

- **Preparation:** Take five minutes to go within and quiet your mind.

- **Instructions:** To create a Declaration of Beauty, choose qualities that light you up or make you feel warm and fuzzy inside. They could be the three words you picked from the "List of Pleasing Qualities" earlier in this chapter; however, for now, stick to two or three words that are descriptive qualities.

Start your Declaration of Beauty one of two ways: Either write, "Who I am is . . ." (try this one first) or "I am . . ." Then, to complete your declaration, insert the two to three descriptive qualities you chose. My personal declaration is, "Who I am is radiant, peaceful and bold."

Be creative. Look within for what speaks to your heart. Your Declaration of Beauty should empower you. It should also inspire you to take actions to align yourself with that declaration. Use it often, and repeat it many times to yourself as you look in the mirror.

After a couple of weeks, you will have a different experience whenever you see your reflection. The best way to commit your declaration to memory is to hum it to yourself on your way to school or work as if it is your very own mantra. Then, when a dump truck of negativity comes your way, remind yourself of your Declaration of Beauty.

Write your Declaration of Beauty here:

"Who I am is: _____,

_____

and _____.

Shift Your Context

When I was studying to become a makeup artist, I was taught that facial beauty comes down to symmetry. The more balance I bring to someone's face, the more likely it is that they will be perceived as attractive.

When I am working on someone's makeup, I never try to change that person's face. For me, the application of makeup should bring out those features that really set a person apart while balancing out any areas that may distract attention from their uniqueness.

Being beautiful is what you experience when you are not distracted from your true nature. Your true nature is one of pure potential and light. *Beauty is who you are.* As you align with your truth, you experience it instead of wish for it.

Instinctively, people are attracted to those who exude physical, mental and emotional balance. While not everyone is born with symmetrical features, everyone can achieve more balance. *Balance is attractive!* Creating a state of balance within your physical body and around your life requires a very high level of consciousness. You must be attentive to your needs in order to sustain the entirety of your well-being—mind, body and spirit.

To experience your true beauty, it is essential to develop a balanced approach to your well-being. It is not enough to focus on the appearance of your body without giving ample attention to your mind and spirit. If these aspects are out of balance, disorders such as bulimia, anorexia, obesity and body dysmorphia may occur.

According to a body image study conducted by Linda Smolak, author of *The Developmental Psychopathology of Eating Disorders,* 80 percent of women are dissatisfied with their appearance, and approximately 7 million women, young and old, struggle with eating disorders because of that dissatisfaction.[1] Conversely, when all three aspects of your well-being are in alignment with the qualities you choose for your Declaration of Beauty, you will feel your beauty to your core. This is a very different feeling than those high highs and low lows that result from recent weight loss or a new hair color. When you spend too much time tending to your physical well-being—instead of approaching your beauty with balance—you fall victim to the woes of this third, classic beauty block.[2]

Once you focus on a balanced approach to your whole body's well-being, you must detach your ideas of beauty from those of *form* and connect them with *qualities* you desire. Lasting happiness with your appearance occurs when you detach from what you think the *form* should look like and instead experience the *qualities* you believe the form represents.

Consider the following ways to shift your context from form to qualities:

LOSING WEIGHT

Form: Size 2, 110 pounds

Qualities: Healthy, energetic, vibrant

STYLISH WARDROBE

Form: Closet full of clothes, 150 pairs of shoes, thousands of accessories

Qualities: Poised, confident, radiant

SUCCESSFUL CAREER

Form: Six-figure salary, corporate car, management of several divisions

Qualities: Powerful, worthy, valued

The form is always specific and rigid by nature; however, particular forms are not linked to the qualities that share the same category. Qualities are experienced in the moment through your actions. By detaching yourself from form and instead connecting to the qualities you desire, you will always be able to experience yourself as beautiful. When you focus on qualities such as being healthy, energetic or vibrant, you tend to make choices that lead you to experience these qualities. Activities such as eating healthier food and moving your body more cease to feel like chores aimed at reaching an arbitrary number. They become simple, yet fulfilling, life choices.

In his book, *The Seven Spiritual Laws of Success,* Deepak Chopra said it best: "Attachment is based on fear and insecurity—and the need for security is based on not knowing the true Self. The source of wealth, of abundance, or of anything in the physical world is the Self; it is the consciousness that knows how to fulfill every need. Everything else is a symbol: cars, houses, bank notes, clothes, airplanes. Symbols are transitory; they come and go. Chasing symbols is like settling for the map instead of the territory."[3]

> *Resist the urge to follow the **trend** and simply be **the real thing.***

When you accept the symbol in place of your true self, your experience creates emptiness. This is why, despite spending more money on beauty products than at any time in history, 80 percent of American women are dissatisfied with their appearance.

Buying products to alter looks clearly does not satisfy women long term. Looks will always change, but when you connect deeply with the qualities you most desire (e.g., love, vitality, acceptance, harmony or peace), they are yours forever.

You cannot obtain your authentic qualities through form. Those things are just representations of the real thing. Magazines and public opinion will always flip-flop from month to month about why brown eyes are in or stripes are a no-no. So, resist the urge to follow the *trend* and simply be the *real thing*.

> *When you are that which you desire, it is permanent and eternal.*

To feel fulfillment in your life, be mindful that form is temporary and fulfillment based on it only lasts as long as the form exists. *When you are that which you desire, it is permanent and eternal.*

Shift Toward Balance

Where do you feel out of balance? Where in your life can you align more with your Declaration of Beauty? Although I have been stressing physical beauty throughout this book, when you feel competent in other areas of your life, you gain confidence. You can extend your Declaration of Beauty into other areas of your life, which will help you feel even more at peace in your skin.

Life continually presents new situations that challenge you to grow and become more of yourself. The goal is not to resist change or avoid challenges but to navigate through challenging situations by staying true to who you are committed to being. The only way I know to stop change is to stop living. This seems like a bleak option! If you find yourself resisting, regretting or bemoaning your growth process, it is once again time to embrace forgiveness, release yourself from these emotions and continue to strive for balance.

As you age and grow in your self-understanding, you will become more adept at identifying what your body needs in its different stages.

When you are committed to achieving real balance in all areas of your life, quick, superficial fixes will not be appealing as you seek out a true state of balance.

Exercise: Journal to Create Balance

- **Location:** A quiet place where you will not be disturbed and where you feel inspired to create and write

- **Materials:** Pen, pencil, computer, journal or spiral notebook

- **Set your timer for:** 15–30 minutes of uninterrupted time

- **Preparation:** Take five minutes to go within and quiet your mind.

- **Instructions:** Pick three areas of your life (for now) and journal about these three areas for the next three to six months. Journaling for this length of time will give you enough material to see your progress over time.

Ask yourself the following questions:

"In what three areas of my life do I want to experience more balance?"

_____

_____

_____

"If I were to experience balance in these three areas of my life, what would it look like or feel like?"

_____

_____

_____

"What can I be doing differently, on a regular basis, that might move me in the direction of what I want to experience?"

_____

_____

_____

_____

"What am I willing to let go of or forgive in order to realize my Declaration of Beauty?"

_____

_____

_____

_____

"What part of the form do I need to let go of to experience what I want?"

_____

_____

_____

_____

CHAPTER 9

Fearless Beauty in Action—
Be It, Do It, Live It!

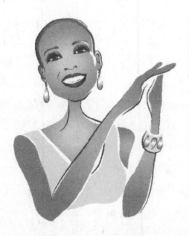

Your time is limited, so don't waste it living someone else's life.
Don't be trapped by dogma—which is living with the results
of other people's thinking. Don't let the noise of other's
opinions drown out your own inner voice. And most important,
have the courage to follow your heart and intuition.
They somehow already know what you truly want to become.
Everything else is secondary.

—Steve Jobs

The Heart and Soul of a Fearless Beauty

Your appearance is not what makes you "you." True, it is generally the first thing people see, but it is rarely what people remember. After meeting you, most people will forget your clothes, hairstyle
and name. It is rare, however, for them to forget your presence. Your
presence is the intangible, magnetic energy that carries influence and

leaves an impression on others you meet. Physical attractiveness may be pleasing to the eye, but it is subjective, and its impact on others pales in comparison to a person's presence.

Presence is the "IT" factor that so many people try to quantify. Presence makes a person attractive to others, even when they are not *traditionally* attractive. It reaches across individual biases concerning appearance and enables a person to define their own influence. The IT factor is unique from person to person. Success, looks, riches, fame or sharp wit may give you access to IT, but they are not IT.

IT cannot be purchased from a store. IT does not accompany a smaller nose or larger breasts. IT stems from how you perceive, treat and carry yourself. IT extends to how you view others and subsequently interact with them. Your physical body is merely a container and, therefore, represents a fraction of how you express your IT factor. Presence encompasses the entirety of your body, mind and spirit. Your individual parts are only expressions of the whole.

> *Presence encompasses the entirety of your body, mind and spirit. Your individual parts are only expressions of the whole.*

Advertisements, movie stars and beauty tips offer ways to mimic a universal IT factor. The beauty establishment uses the media to convince you that you are better off if you employ their beauty codes and rituals because they profit when you follow along. Their focus on physical aspects, however, makes their presentation of IT a fabrication. The IT factor results from a person's harmony from the inside out.

There is nothing essentially wrong with the beauty industry's way of thinking. Their products may enhance your appearance and even inspire you. You simply cannot allow such things to consume you. Using beauty products as a replacement for empowering the real you to shine will only enhance one aspect of your beauty, resulting in those feelings of temporary fulfillment we talked about in Chapter 1. Alternatively, connecting to qualities that you want to embody is the foundation for generating your IT factor.

You carry within you the secret to your Fearless Beauty!

Committing yourself to live true to your Declaration of Beauty builds muscles of confidence around your true expression. Confident self-expression translates into real presence, real beauty—Fearless Beauty.

Fearless Beauty is the freedom to express who you are to the world—not who you think others expect you to be or who you think you "should" be. The Fearless Beauty knows herself and is committed to living a life true to what is in her heart and soul.

The bold expression of your Declaration of Beauty and your heart's authenticity in the pursuit of that declaration transcend physical appearance. They foster an environment in which your presence prevails.

IT is irresistible to others.

IT is pure.

IT is beautiful.

> *Fearless Beauty is the freedom to express who you are to the world—not who you think others expect you to be or who you think you "should" be.*

When your inner radiance shines brightly enough to become visible to everyone around you—regardless of how you dress it, press it, plump it, lift it, fix it or tuck it—you have IT!

You must recognize and nurture your IT factor first. Others will follow suit.

Achieving Your IT Factor

The goal of this book is to help you own the power of your Fearless Beauty. By now, I hope you recognize how your Fearless Beauty is far more than your physical appearance. It is all of you. Recognizing your physical beauty and being confident in its existence requires an inside-out job. You must constantly tend to your emotional, spiritual and physical well-being to realize your true beauty. As you tend to these areas with balance and witness the positive changes within you, you build the confidence necessary to declare yourself as beautiful.

You can apply the six-step process laid out in this book to any area of your life. Following is a recap of the entire process you just advanced through in this book. The final step is not included in the summary below. Instead, Chapter 10 discusses the sixth stage of the process in its entirety. This beauty ritual will give you the tools to internalize your Declaration of Beauty at the physical, mental and spiritual levels. It is designed to progress you through your blocks quickly while helping you embody, with every fiber of your being, the possibility of what you most desire.

STEP ONE
Indentify What You Want and Why

Express what you want with language. This is the foundation of creation. Whether you write it on a piece of paper or record it with your voice recorder, language creates your physical reality. Initially, your desires may not be clear to you. This is why I suggest you develop the habit of journaling. As you might have noticed, each of the exercises in the book has required some form of written response. By simply completing these exercises, you have become accustomed to a form of journaling. Apply this to your daily life. Inspiration for what you want in your life comes to mind all the time. Make a note of any inspiring observations or conversations that arise throughout your day. By capturing the stimuli that motivate you, you clarify your deepest wants.

In Chapter 1, you answered a series of questions concerning your definition of beauty and why beauty is important to you. You can apply this sort of questioning to any area of your life. Whether contemplating a particular career that you want to pursue or the type of lifestyle you want to embody, asking yourself the *Who, What, When, Where* and, most importantly, *Why* regarding your situation will shed light on your true desires.

Shortly after I committed to writing this book, I attended Maria

Shriver's Women's Conference in Long Beach, CA. I was way up in the bleachers with my roommate, amazed at the energy and beauty of all the women—at least 10,000—that filled that convention center. The Dalai Lama came to the stage to speak. As Maria Shriver interviewed the Dalai Lama, I imagined that I had captivated the attention of the entire audience, as he had. My vision was so vivid and powerful that I wrote it down in my journal, and I refer back to it often. Since then, the desire behind that vision has crystallized by writing this book and journaling about other observations I have made. Journaling has enabled me to better understand and satisfy my desire to help others. The possibilities of what journaling might do for you are endless.

STEP TWO
Distinguish What Blocks Are in Your Way

In Chapter 1, I specifically identified three blocks that prevent women from feeling beautiful. I believe these same three blocks obstruct most things we want in our lives. Regardless of what we desire, the only real obstacles that restrict us from pursuing our desires are those that we create. To identify which blocks keep you in a holding pattern, start by looking at your behavior toward those things you desire. Then, refer back to Chapters 2 and 3 to determine how your Herstory (your interpretation of your past) has defined what is possible in this area of your life. Understanding how your past restricts your potential enables you to identify the self-sabotaging statements your Delusional Diva makes whenever you go outside of your element to attempt something that feels a bit unsafe.

Write out your story, then work to release all of the emotional charges that you have built up around it. Repeatedly tell your story until you realize that it is just a story. If you do not have a lot of emotional baggage attached to your story, you may simply need to let it go and move to step three.

STEP THREE
Make Room for What You Want

Forgiveness offers freedom from your past. It also frees you from the resulting beliefs that try to define what you can, or cannot, accomplish. When freedom is present, anything—and I do mean *anything*—is possible. Without the presence of your past constraints, you will recognize and experience the Fearless Beauty that you are, and your actions will become more consistent with what you desire most.

Making forgiveness part of your daily life will allow you to move through life's challenges faster and with an open heart. You will find that those circumstances that trigger negative reactions within you occur less frequently. You will get over them much faster as well. The more you offer forgiveness, the less likely you are to harbor feelings that stand in the way of realizing your wants.

STEP FOUR
Eliminate Comparisons

Unfair comparisons may include comparisons with other people or yourself. If you discover new wants that you are unfamiliar with, your knowledge base and new muscles in that area will require time to develop. It is unfair to compare yourself to others who are further along than you are, especially when you have not traveled down the same path as they have. Everyone has to start somewhere. Eliminating comparisons will allow you to proceed at your own pace. Instead of comparing yourself with others who have more experience, it is more beneficial to seek out mentors from which to learn. This will help you build your muscles stronger, faster. Moreover, it will enable you to avoid some of the pitfalls others have encountered in their pursuit of similar desires.

It is also important to avoid comparing your current self with your achievements or failures. You cannot depend on your past to propel you into a new future. Use your past to identify the behaviors and patterns that are not conducive to what you want and also those that are beneficial and should remain in your life. Do not allow your past to use you by creating additional judgment and limitations. In other words, learn what you need to learn from your past in order to create your desired future. Do not become stuck comparing the you of today to the you of your past. Honing your ability to use comparisons constructively will become easier if you keep a record of those things you desire to experience more often. This enables you to constantly clarify your wants and modify your actions accordingly.

STEP FIVE
Create a Declaration

Create a declaration of what you want based on the qualities that you want to experience. Here is the caveat to that statement: Without action, a declaration is nothing but empty words. In addition, action without clear intention is like a hamster running on a wheel—a lot is happening, but nothing is accomplished. Action sets your declaration in motion, and intention keeps it moving in your desired direction.

A declaration, similar to an affirmation, is a tool that works on your belief system over time. Use it to reinvigorate your desire to take action to achieve whatever is most important to you. Your declaration should inspire you. If it does not, change it. If you feel like nothing is drawing you toward the positive changes your life needs, you may be hanging on to resentment or limiting beliefs from your past. Revisit Chapter 2 to determine what prevents you from pursuing your desires. Then, bring forgiveness to that remnant of your past.

With a strong declaration guiding you, determine what actions are necessary for you to create the new reality you desire. Begin by looking within yourself. Let your intuition guide you as you choose your course of action.

The Beauty Ritual

A Fearless Beauty's movement is always inspired by her heart's desires, not her fears. Your desire to become radiant, confident and sexy requires action. Consistent, daily action focused on your holistic well-being is the cornerstone for moving through your journey to become a Fearless Beauty.

Your regular old beauty regimen aimed at maintaining your physical body will not cut it! Now we arrive at the key for coming full circle to discover your Fearless Beauty. You must create holistic wellness by adopting a daily beauty ritual that engages your body, mind and spirit. This balance in your beauty ritual will lead you to appreciate yourself from the inside out. You will feel comfortable and confident in your skin. Achieving balance in your body's wellness and finding your unique beauty will take time. However, incorporating body movement, meditation and journaling into your daily routine will help you to embody the qualities you identify as important to you.

Qualities are, in essence, a state of being. Your being needs to embody your Declaration of Beauty for it to become a reality. Remember we said that without action your declaration is just words? Your beauty ritual is the vehicle—the action—that will infuse your Declaration of Beauty into your body, mind and spirit. It will require practice to determine which techniques in relation to your body, mind and spirit are best suited for you. I encourage you to try different modalities in order to find what works.

In the next chapter, I will reveal the specific activities that I employ in order to embody my Declaration of Beauty. My hope is that they will lead you to a deeper understanding of the connection between your body, mind and spirit. They should also serve as a stepping-stone to a wider range of possible beauty rituals that can empower you to experience more of yourself.

Regardless of where you are in your exploration to find—or refine—your perfect beauty ritual, always "mind the gap" (as they say in England, when entering or exiting their subway trains). The gap is the space between where you are and where you want to be. Give yourself compassion during the transition from one place to the next.

I know this can be difficult, especially if you prefer to keep a consistent schedule and suddenly the bottom slips right out from underneath you. One missed day can lead to another. Then, all of a sudden, you have skipped a whole week—or even months—of making time for yourself. Don't let discouragement or self-judgment keep you from choosing to reset and start again. Give yourself grace and then choose to reset and start again.

If you find yourself *constantly* in fits and starts with regard to your daily beauty ritual, maybe it's time to reevaluate your schedule. Perhaps the time slot you've set aside for your practice isn't practical and moving it to a different time of day (or evening) would go a long way toward helping you create a consistent practice.

Many people also find that accountability is a great help in achieving their goals. Share your intention with a friend and arrange a regular time to check in. Better yet, invite a friend to join you on your journey to Fearless Beauty and keep one another accountable. Having a companion on this path doubles the fun and the rewards as you share your celebration of growth along the way.

Your daily beauty ritual will keep you on your desired path. It will continuously aid you in releasing toxins, such as fear, from your physical body, and it will also build new muscles that help you embody your goals and reinforce your confidence in your intuition.

But it won't deliver any of these benefits without one thing—consistent action. You wouldn't dream of brushing your teeth once in a while and expect to have good dental health, right? You know that a consistent habit of flossing and brushing will keep your gums and teeth healthy, so you do it day in and day out (I hope), even on the days when you don't necessarily feel enthused about it. It's simply a non-negotiable activity that you've carved into your daily routine because it is good for you.

Your daily beauty ritual is no different. Even during times when you don't feel like anything significant is happening as a result of your practice, remember that your consistent investment in yourself is its own reward. It is a tangible way to communicate to yourself, "I am important and worth caring for." Trust me—with consistent action will come confidence, serenity and a sense of balance that will motivate you to make your daily beauty ritual one of the non-negotiables in your life.

I would be lying if I didn't admit to letting my daily beauty ritual slide from time to time. Each time I allow large chunks of time to pass without doing my beauty ritual, I notice that doubt and fear creep into my mind. Such lapses in time away from my beauty ritual even made writing this book take far longer than I ever anticipated. Once I returned to my daily practices, however, my vision and my desire to inspire *beauty* took center stage again.

Creating a beauty ritual will help you eliminate your fears. More importantly, it will build up your confidence, enabling you to move forward in the face of those fears. This entire process will demonstrate that fear is not real. Only your thoughts about it are real. There is nothing on this planet that you cannot achieve or overcome. Once you understand this to the core of your existence, the world is your playground.

Motivation to Create and Maintain a Daily Beauty Ritual

If your life is anything like mine, you are running non-stop from the time you wake up until the minute you lay your head down to go to sleep. I realize that adding a beauty ritual to your schedule might seem like adding another mere task to your to-do list. On the contrary, setting aside this time for yourself will prove to boost your confidence and increase your productivity throughout your day.

Finding time to devote to your daily beauty ritual is just as important as making dinner, organizing your next board meeting or spending time with family. Whenever I don't feel like I have enough time to take care of me, I lean on the words of wisdom in my friend Erika's story. (She is not just a breast cancer survivor; she thrives.)

The day after I had my first surgery, while I was at home resting, I received a phone call from one of my long-time clients. Initially, I thought, "Oh wow, how thoughtful of her," which is what made me answer my phone in the first place even though I was physically drained. The conversation started with small talk, with her asking me how I was doing. When I replied, "I'm hanging in there," not even a second lapsed after I finished my sentence before she said, "Girl, I know you just had surgery, but can you do my hair on Friday?" Immediately, and without much thought, I said, "NO!" This is something I had never done before. In that instance, I realized she didn't value me or what I was going through. She just wanted her needs met. It was in that moment that I realized I had to put a value on my own life.

For so long, I took care of everyone else's needs. Even when I look at my accomplishments, I can see that I did them because it was what others expected of me. I loved to make others happy, so I carried their junk on my back until their burdens wore me down. Cancer was a backhand blessing for me. It gave me clarity to put myself first. If I don't take care of me, how will I ever be able to take care of anyone else?

Not long after, during my recovery, I looked in the mirror and saw an amazing woman who needed to be cared for by me. Me! That realization made me feel more beautiful than I ever had before. When I put a value on my life and the time I need for me, I became more powerful than ever before. Now, I embrace everything about myself and keep falling in love with the person that I see and the person I continue to grow into.

Life happens, and you will find that everything from considerable catastrophes to annoying inconveniences will conspire to distract you from keeping your commitment to yourself. Because you may not recognize the value your daily beauty ritual adds to your life, you may be inclined to skip it on busy days. It is only through your consistent practice of this ritual, however, that you will discover how necessary it is. Stick with your ritual and always have your "why" front and center to keep you inspired. You should treat this time with the utmost importance.

Beware! The moment your daily practice starts working, your Delusional Diva will kick in and try to convince you that you no longer need to make time for yourself. To prevent this from happening, I suggest that you do not create your daily beauty ritual to achieve a particular result. Doing so could allow you to stop your ritual once you have achieved that goal. Think of your beauty ritual as something that is just as necessary as brushing your teeth. This perspective will help your ritual become a lifelong practice.

Making time for your beauty ritual does not have to be difficult, especially if you go about it strategically. Start by drawing up a timetable for yourself. It doesn't have to be exact. Just sketch a simple schedule of a typical week on a piece of paper. List all of your regular activities. These may include going to work (include travel time), taking the kids to school, shopping on a Saturday afternoon or bowling in the league on Tuesdays. Do not forget to include the time you go to bed each evening. It is important to block out time for that as well.

When you have written all of your regular events on your schedule, make a list of tasks that you should do regularly but might, occasionally, miss. These tasks might include filing paperwork, paying bills and writing emails. By allocating time for these tasks, you create a complete picture of how your time is spent. Since these activities could vary from week to week, you may want to create a block of two or three hours on your timetable to catch up on these tasks before they get out of hand. After you have included this on your schedule, look at your timetable.

You might find that you have more time available than you originally thought. If this is the case, perhaps you spend more time surfing the internet or watching TV than you realize. On the other hand, you may be doing things for other people that they can do for themselves. If you have plenty of blank spaces on your timetable but cannot account for them, keep a diary of all your activities for a week. Note how much time you spend on each activity. Shopping might prove to take twice as long as you thought. You might also find that you forgot to include a regular task in your schedule. A diary will help you spot these things and plug the holes in your timetable.

When you have done this, study your timetable and see what time you have left. It is very likely that you will have some spare slots to devote to your beauty ritual. Nevertheless, if your timetable is packed, then you should look carefully at what uses up all of your time. If it is work, do another timetable for work and prioritize all of your work tasks within it. If you cannot fit all of those tasks in, you have identified a problem—you are overworked! Get help, and delegate the tasks you do not need to do. Sometimes, all you need to do is clearly communicate your desires with others. If your requests are ignored, however, you may have to be firm. Find what works for you and be flexible with the time. But do not skip out on your daily beauty ritual.

Exercise: Finding Time for You

- **Location:** A quiet place where you will not be disturbed

- **Materials:** A pencil or pen and the *Finding Time for Me Worksheet*

- **Set your timer for:** 30 minutes of uninterrupted time

- **Preparation:** Take five minutes to go within and quiet your mind.

- **Instructions:** Use the following worksheet to map out your current schedule. Then, plot out times on each day of the week where you will make time just for you.

FINDING TIME FOR ME WORKSHEET							
	SUNDAY	MONDAY	TUESDAY	WEDNESDAY	THURSDAY	FRIDAY	SATURDAY
5 am							
6 am							
7 am							
8 am							
9 am							
10 am							
11 am							
12 pm							
1 pm							
2 pm							
3 pm							
4 pm							

	SUNDAY	MONDAY	TUESDAY	WEDNESDAY	THURSDAY	FRIDAY	SATURDAY
5 pm							
6 pm							
7 pm							
8 pm							
9 pm							
10 pm							
11 pm							
12 am							
1 am							
2 am							
3 am							
4 am							

CHAPTER 10

Fearless Beauty Ritual—
Putting It All Together

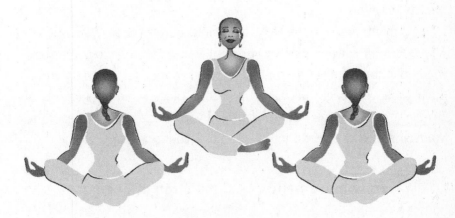

Love life, engage in it, give it all you've got.
Love it with a passion, because life truly does give back,
many times over, what you put into it.

—Maya Angelou

STEP SIX
Create Your Fearless Beauty Ritual

Now that you have your schedule laid out in front of you, it is time to decide where your daily beauty ritual will fit in. Even if you find it works best to alternate the time of day you practice your ritual, I encourage you, if possible, to schedule the same *amount* of time every day. Whatever your schedule looks like, make a daily habit of blocking out time just for you. This will help you break the third block that keeps women from feeling beautiful—finding time to care for their holistic well-being.

Your beauty ritual will consist of three separate activities: body movement, meditation and journaling. All of these activities can be completed within an hour. (If time is tight, these tasks can be finished in 40 to 45 minutes.) By doing these three activities on a daily basis, you will find you have more clarity and focus throughout your day. You will also develop a more balanced perspective of your beauty than just your physical body.

As I mentioned in the very beginning of the book, you are all-knowing. Your specific journey will lead you to those actions that best feed your soul during the time set aside for your daily beauty ritual. Each time you begin your beauty ritual, place your Declaration of Beauty in front of you. Feel free to read your Declaration of Beauty to yourself as a way of honoring yourself and your practice.

Body Movement: The Circulation of Energy

Your body is the container that holds your IT factor, so it is vitally important to keep it moving. At the very minimum, your body movement should circulate your energy. The circulation of energy through your body will help with two things. First, body movement helps eliminate toxins. These can come in physical forms, such as unused food, or emotional forms, such as fear, resentment and anger. Body movement also builds a stronger body, immune system, muscles, etc. By strengthening the physical construction of your body,

When you allow your body, mind and spirit to connect, you create a powerful space in which you can achieve all of your desires.

your body's potential expands. You will feel more capable. When you allow your body, mind and spirit to connect, you create a powerful space in which you can achieve all of your desires.

Years ago, I worked at a women-only fitness facility. I started as an aerobics instructor, moved into sales and eventually worked my way up to a position of management over several clubs. As I grew with the company, I never stopped teaching aerobics. It remained the most inspiring part of my day.

The capabilities of the women who stepped onto that aerobics floor varied. Some had no coordination. Others were just starting to exercise for the first time. For the women who stayed with me, I witnessed transformations in their physical bodies as well as in their attitudes and confidence. They often approached me, bragging about how they finally learned to use their arms in coordination with their feet. Some remarked that they were proud to be able to make it all the way to the end of class. Each victory was a personal breakthrough. They experienced an enormous, unexpected amount of reverence for what their bodies were capable of.

Before I give you the specifics about the bodywork in my beauty ritual, I want to make a disclaimer: Do not start any new exercises without first consulting your physician to be sure that you can do each of these poses without jeopardizing yourself in anyway. After consulting your physician, I also encourage you to find a physical exercise that you are comfortable incorporating into your schedule three days a week. Try to find an exercise that increases your heart rate for at least one hour on those days. This exercise should be included in your schedule in addition to the normal body movement portion of your daily beauty ritual.

Although the body movement I am proposing here is a beginner series of yoga poses, I strongly advise you to consult with your physician before moving forward with this body movement. It is important to be certain that you are building your body up, not tearing it down. I specifically chose this body movement option to help you listen to your body on a deep level. It will support you as you carry out the other exercise you choose to do three times a week.

Yoga is an ancient tradition that has been modified from region to region; however, it is best known for its historical ties to India. Many of the poses are written in Sanskrit. Sun Salutations, called *surya namaskar* in Sanskrit, are designed to generate heat in order to cleanse your body and mind. It is a form of moving meditation. This flowing series of poses honors the life-sustaining energy of the sun as well as your own life force. The Sun Salutation gets your heart pumping, stretches your muscles, increases circulation and takes your body through a full range of motion.

Exercise: Body Movement—Sun Salutation

- **Location:** A quiet place where you will not be disturbed

- **Materials:** Yoga mat, comfortable clothing

- **Set your timer for:** 15–20 minutes of uninterrupted time

- **Preparation:** Warm up your body by marching in place, doing jumping jacks or rotating your joints back and forth.

- **Instructions:** There are 12 different postures in this series, each of which I will go over with you in detail. When combined in sequence, these postures form the Sun Salutation.

The Sun Salutation

1. The Sun Salutation begins in a standing position with your feet side by side at the front edge of your exercise mat. Bend your arms at the elbows, and place your palms together in front of your chest. Relax in this pose for a moment or two, and then begin to inhale. This standing pose helps to ground you to the earth, builds body awareness within you and helps you find your center.

2. As you *continue* to draw in that breath, move into the second position: Raise your arms high overhead and lean backward, arching your spine slightly.

3. Then—while you exhale—bend forward from the waist and drop

your head toward your knees. (Your knees should not bend.) Allow the weight of your torso to help you rest your hands on the floor in front of your feet. Do not worry if you are not able to touch the floor in front of you. Just imagine that as your intention. This forward bend stretches your hamstrings and elongates your spine.

4. The fourth position is also performed while inhaling. Keeping your hands on the floor, bend both of your knees and stretch your left leg, then your right leg, out behind you. This is called the plank position. Then, bend your knees slightly, so that both of your knees are resting on the floor. Flex your toes under on the yoga mat for a good grip. Then, arch your back, and look upward. This halfway lift also elongates your spine and cleanses your digestive system.

5. Next, exhale as you straighten your right leg and move your left leg. Push your buttocks up to form an inverted "V" with your body, and let your head hang loosely between your arms. Your back—from shoulders to hips—should be as straight as possible. Pull your stomach in toward the spine, and try to press your heels flat against the floor.

6. As you move into the next pose, you will need to hold your breath. Bend both of your arms at the elbows, and carefully lower your body to the floor, with contact points at the forehead, chest, hands and knees. Keep your pelvis, abdomen and thighs raised, and press your chin into the hollow at the base of your throat. Lowering from plank into four-legged staff pose requires core and arm strength. Feel free to modify this pose as you develop these muscles. You may lower your knees, chest and chin to modify the position. Plank and four-limb staff poses engage the muscles in your arms, shoulders, chest and abdomen.

7. Now, as you inhale, lower your pelvis and legs onto the floor, straighten your arms, arch your back and let your head tilt backward. This upward-facing dog position stretches your upper body as it opens your chest and frees your breathing.

8. With this position, you begin to reverse the cycle and move back toward the starting point. As you exhale, thrust your hips high, forming an inverted "V" again. Downward-facing dog works muscles in your entire body and calms your nervous system.

9. Next, inhale and move your right leg forward until that foot rests on the floor between your hands. Extend your left leg back, touching the floor with your knee. Also, lean your head back. (You will notice that this pose is an alternate-leg version of No. 4.)

10. As you exhale, bring the left foot up beside the right. Then, straighten both legs and drop your torso until your head approaches your knees again.

11. Inhale and stand up straight as you stretch your arms high overhead.

12. On the last exhale, bring your hands back together in front of your chest to pay a final homage to the morning sun. Breathe freely for a few moments.

You can do as many sets of these poses as you like, but always try to do at least two sets to bring balance to both sides of your body. The Sun Salutation is an excellent way to jump-start your beauty ritual. Spend 15–20 minutes on your body movement. This should consist of 10–15 minutes of Sun Salutations, followed by five minutes resting on your mat. Rest by lying on your back with your heels touching, your toes falling away from your body and your arms near your side.

Embracing your body in a way that connects it with your mind and spirit helps you think of your body as more than just an object to dress up. How you deal with your body is a metaphor for other areas of importance. It is emblematic of calming yourself with proper breathing, moving through cravings or obsessing about your looks.

Meditation: Calming the Mind, Activating the Spirit

In Chapter 1, we talked about meditation at greater length. Please revisit that section to remind yourself of the benefits of meditation and how to approach it. If you are able to do each of your beauty rituals back to back to back, I suggest that you sit up from your resting position (after yoga) and proceed directly into your meditation. It might be helpful to have an alarm near you to help you stick to a specific timeframe. Set it to ring approximately 20–30 minutes from the start of your meditation. Turn off your ringer and all other cell phone notifications so that you are not interrupted during your meditation. Your phone should have an option that allows only the alarm to sound, but nothing else.

Use your allotted time to go within and be silent. You might feel very uncomfortable during the first week or first month of your practice. You might find, as I did, that your mind is racing constantly during your time of silence. You may even think that your meditation isn't working. Nevertheless, any effort to sit in silence *is* working. It only stops working if you give up, so resist the urge to throw in the towel.

Here are three different ways in which you can meditate if you find that sitting in stillness is not helping you to quiet your mind.

• Use a mantra or repeat a word that soothes and relaxes your mind, such as *ooommm, rummmmmm* or *aaaaahhhhh oooommmm*. Let it vibrate in your mouth as you inhale and exhale.

• Use breath and visualization. See your breath come into your body as you witness your chest and belly rise. Then, watch it move out of your body as your belly and chest collapse.

• Allow your thoughts to enter your head. Acknowledge the thoughts, and release them with your next breath. Do not try to stop or resist these thoughts because what you resist persists.

Over time, you will find that your thoughts will quiet, and you will enter deep stillness with greater ease. Be sure to approach meditation with compassion and patience if this is completely new to you. Remember, it takes time to build new muscles.

Journaling: Expand and Release

You can round out your daily beauty ritual with a journaling exercise to capture any insights you may have had during this time. Journaling on a regular basis is a powerful tool to help you clarify your thoughts and feelings. By doing so, you gain valuable self-knowledge that helps to create balance in your life. Journaling can also guide you through stressful events and allow you to understand your thought process and hidden desires. Once you have been journaling for a while, you can look back at your entries to find gaps or patterns that may lead you to more balance and greater happiness.

There is no right way to journal. You can keep a journal on your computer, in a spiral notebook or in a fancy keepsake book with blank pages. You can keep a specific journal, such as a gratitude journal, a dream journal or an observation journal as the basis for what you express during your journaling. On the other hand, you can also allow yourself to write in a free flow manner every time you put your pen to paper.

The length of time you spend journaling—2, 5, 10, 15 or 30 minutes a day—is up to you. Spending a small amount of time journaling is better than not doing it at all. I tend to journal a second time at night, which helps me purge my thoughts from the day so I can get a good night's rest.

It is important to get in the habit of writing out your thoughts and expressing yourself authentically without filters. Here are more examples of journaling exercises:

Journal Your Wants and Desires

Here are a few questions that you may want to consider when journaling on a regular basis:

1. What is it that I really want?

2. When would I like this to happen?

3. What is the feeling I want to experience from having or doing this in my life? Make a list.

4. Why is this important to me?

Journal to Forgive

Forgiveness is a choice that offers great rewards. To make forgiveness easier, journal daily about a current situation that you desire to let go of. After writing one of the statements below in your journal, let whatever flows from your heart and head spill out on the paper. If you find yourself completely freed up in all of your relationships, use these statements to offer forgiveness and compassion to worldly issues that emotionally bind you:

1. I release the emotional ties that bind me to this person or situation because . . .

2. I completely forgive this person or situation because . . .

3. I am grateful for this person and situation because . . .

Your answers to these questions will build a case for you to forgive. Once you understand why it is necessary to offer forgiveness to this person or situation, you must take action. Visit Chapter 5's Exercise: Forgive and Let Go of Past Hurts, offer your love, compassion and forgiveness to this person or situation and keep moving in the direction of your desires.

Honoring Your Season of Life

If you are reading about the daily beauty ritual and thinking, "If this is what I have to do to be beautiful inside and out, I will NEVER be beautiful! There's no way I can possibly carve out this kind of time right now." Maybe you've just started a new job, and the learning curve has you working 10- to 12-hour days. You are doing good just to get a decent night's sleep. Or maybe you are a young mom whose idea of time alone is to sneak away to the bathroom by yourself for five minutes.

There are seasons of life when your daily beauty ritual will need to be adjusted in order to remain consistent. Do not give up on your practice during these seasons. In fact, it is during the most demanding times of our lives that our daily beauty ritual becomes a lifeline to keep us connected to who we are so that we do not begin to define our-selves merely by what we do. Our daily beauty ritual keeps us centered and helps sustain us through seasons that can potentially leave us drained both physically and emotionally.

If you are a young mom, maybe your movement will involve playing with your little ones at the park or plugging in a yoga DVD at home. And, yes, they might decide to climb on your back during one of your poses—that is your opportunity to practice gratitude for the great priv-ilege of being their mom. Can you arrange for a friend, your spouse or another mom to watch the kids for an hour each week? This could be your special time that you look forward to all week when you are able to engage in movement, meditation and journaling. For your daily rit-ual, see if you can carve out 10 minutes during naptime or before they wake up. You can alternate between journaling, meditation and move-ment each day. If you are a nursing mom, try spending that time in meditation. Look within yourself for the wisdom to create a practical daily beauty ritual that makes sense in this special season of life.

If the current demands of your job leave you little time for yourself, can you use a portion of your break or lunchtime to engage in one aspect of your beauty ritual? Again, maybe you will need to alternate the activities of your routine during the week and set aside an hour on the weekend to practice all three components—movement, meditation and journaling.

You've heard the saying, "Where there is a will, there is a way." If your will, or intention, is to recognize and embrace your Fearless Beauty, you will discover a way to engage in your daily beauty ritual. It just takes some creativity, the willingness to give yourself grace, and the intention to make it happen.

My Wishes for You

My wish is that you become—if you are not already—one of the 2 percent of women who use the word "beautiful" to describe themselves. I hope becoming a Fearless Beauty leads you to share your beauty secrets with the other 98 percent who do not describe themselves as beautiful. Collectively, we can change this statistic to read, "Ninety-eight percent of women use the word 'beautiful' to describe themselves!"

My wish is that you will face life's challenges with an open heart and that you will view each challenge as an opportunity for you to become more of yourself. Keep in mind that the goal is not to stop change or avoid challenges. Instead, it is to navigate through them, staying true to the person you are committed to being. If you find yourself resisting, regretting or bemoaning the process of growth, it is time to embrace forgiveness again and release yourself from these emotions.

Allow yourself to unfold with grace, ease and wisdom from within.

My wish is that you will experience the profound wisdom of your soul and do the work on this planet that you came here to do.

My wish is that you will catch a vision so large that it scares the pants off of you . . . and that you will think back to this book and remember that *fear is only an illusion.*

My wish is that you will make your light known to yourself and to others. Your gift is necessary on this planet at this particular time in our human evolution.

Allow yourself to unfold with grace, ease and wisdom from within. Embrace all of life's challenges, and welcome the changes to your physical beauty.

If you do this, your Fearless Beauty will shine even brighter with every passing year.

References

Chapter 1

1. Richard Perez-Pena, The New York Times, "U.S. Bachelor Degree Rate Passes Milestone" February 23, 2012

2. Ekaterina Walter, "The top 30 stats you need to know when marketing to women" http://thenextweb.com January 24, 2012

3. The American Society for Aesthetic Plastic Surgery, "Cosmetic Plastic Surgery Research: Statistics and Trends for 2001–2010" (www.cosmeticplastic surgerystatistics.com/statistics.html#2007-New).

4. Hoovers.com. "Cosmetics, Beauty Supply and Perfume Stores Industry Overview" (www.hoovers.com/cosmetics,-beauty-supply,-and-perfume-stores/—ID__294—/free-ind-fr-profile-basic.xhtml). "In 2010 US consumer spend on beauty products recovered slowly after the losses of 2009, posting a total value of $59bn, a figure that is predicted to rise slowly to 62.0bn by the end of 2015." "Key cosmetic trends to fight the economic doldrums." "Although market researcher Demeter Group is predicting tougher times for the US cosmetics industry in the second half of 2011, there are a handful of key industry trends that are expected to cushion the blow." www.cosmeticsdesign.com/Market-Trends/Key-cosmetic-trends-to-fight-the-economic-doldrums (www.cosmetics design.com/Market-Trends/ Key-cosmetic-trends-to-fight-the-economic-doldrums).

5. Dr. Nancy Etcoff, et al., "The Real Truth About Beauty: A Global Report," September 2004, p. 9 (www.strategyone.com/documents/dove_white_paper _final.pdf).

6. Naomi Wolf, *The Beauty Myth* (New York: HarperCollins Publishers, Inc., 2002), p. 10; Center for American Women and Politics, Eagleton Institute of Politics (http://www.cawp.rutgers.edu).

7. Jennifer Pozner, *Reality Bites Back* (Berkeley, CA: Seal Press, 2010), p. 97.

8. YWCA, *Beauty at Any Cost: The Consequences of America's Beauty Obsession on Women & Girls* (New York: YWCA USA, August 2008), p. 4 (www.ywca .org/atf/cf/%7B711d5519-9e3c-4362-b753 ad138b 5d352c%7D/BEAUTY-AT-ANY-COST.PDF); cited from [14] "Disordered Eating Is Widespread among U.S. Women."Online Survey by SELF magazine in partnership with the University of North Carolina at Chapel Hill. 2008. U.S. Department of Health & Human Services. National Women's Health Information Center.

9. Note 17, supra; cited from [21] 'National Eating Disorders Association Fact Sheet' (May 2008) (www.nationaleatingdisorders.org/

10. Note 17, supra; cited from [17] 'Disordered Eating Is Widespread among U.S. Women.' Online Survey by SELF magazine in partnership with the University of North Carolina at Chapel Hill. 2008. U.S. Department of Health & Human Services. National Women's Health Information Center (www.womenshealth .gov/news/english/614866.htm) (online poll of more than 4,000 women between the ages of 25 and 45)."

11. Note 17, supra; cited from [20] American Lung Association. 'Women and Smoking Fact Sheet' (2007) (www.lungusa.org/site/c.dvLUK9O0E/b.33572/ k.985F/Women_and_Smoking_Fact_Sheet.htm).

12. Deepak Chopra, *The Seven Spiritual Laws of Success* (San Rafael, CA, Amber-Allen Publishing, 1994), p. 2.

13. Marianne Williamson, *A Return to Love: Reflections on the Principles of "A Course in Miracles"* (New York, NY: HarperCollins Publishers, Inc., 1992), p. 191.

14. www.blogher.com/would-american-economy-collapse-if-women-stopped-hating-their-natural-appearance-look-makeup

Chapter 2

1. Dr. Nancy Etcoff, et al., "The Real Truth About Beauty: A Global Report," September 2004, p. 9 (www.strategyone.com/documents/dove_white_paper_final.pdf).

2. http://en.wikipedia.org/wiki/Self-image

Chapter 3

1. Smolak, L. (1996). National Eating Disorders Association/Next Door Neighbors Puppet Guide Book.

2. Dan Miller, *No More Mondays* (New York: Doubleday Publishing, 2008), p. 63.

Chapter 5

1. J. North, "The 'Ideal' of Forgiveness: A Philosopher's Exploration" in *Exploring Forgiveness,* edited by Enright & North, pp. 20-21.

2. Mayo Clinic, "Learning To Forgive May Improve Well-Being," 2008.

3. "Forgive and Forget" (www.webmd.com/balance/guide/forgive-forget?page=2).

4. Louise L. Hay, *You Can Heal Your Life* (Santa Monica, CA: Hay House Publishing, 2004), p. 221.

Chapter 6

1. Deepak Chopra, *The Seven Spiritual Laws of Success* (San Rafael, CA: Amber-Allen Publishing, 1994).

Chapter 7

1. Used with permission from a recorded telephone conversation.

Chapter 8

1. Smolak, L. (1996). National Eating Disorders Association/Next Door Neighbors Puppet Guide Book.

2. Ibid.

3. Deepak Chopra, *The Seven Spiritual Laws of Success* (San Rafael, CA: Amber-Allen Publishing, 1994), p. 84.

Index

About the Author

KENETIA LEE, Beauty Activist, Author, Makeup Artist
www.beautyactivist.com

Kenetia Lee is one of today's leading authorities on beauty empowerment. As a highly respected professional makeup artist, author, personal coach, and speaker, Kenetia is living her life purpose to empower women all over the world to embrace the unique beauty that lives within them.

From the everyday women who sat in her makeup chair to stunning models and famous celebrities, Kenetia has encountered face to face the damaging effects that result from a negative self-image. These experiences, coupled with her own personal story, moved Kenetia to a lifelong mission—to transform women from the inside out, to lift them from the darkness of self-deprecation and to inspire them to celebrate the artistry of each brilliant feature they possess. Passionately committed to helping women live boldly and beautifully, Kenetia encourages women all over the country to appreciate themselves and embrace their beauty fearlessly.

Kenetia is a highly sought-after Red Carpet Makeup Artist and has had the honor of working intimately with beautiful women at the Academy Awards, the Golden Globe Awards, the Grammy Awards, the Victoria's Secret Fashion Show, and Teen Vogue Fashion LIVE to name a few. As a public speaker and spokesperson, she has worked with Revlon, Covergirl, Mark Cosmetics, The Miss Universe Organization, Step Up Women's Network, and numerous other national organizations. Kenetia has regularly appeared on television shows such as ABC's *Eyewitness News Sunday Morning,* WB's *Good Day Arizona,* WB's *Flix & Pix Detroit,* and CW's *Extra!* Kenetia is also a featured columnist in publications such as *InStyle, The Las Vegas Review,* and *The Los Angeles Sentinel.*

In **Fearless Beauty 360°,** Kenetia presents a practical yet powerful blueprint for physical well-being, mental clarity, and spiritual fulfillment. Her timely message gives women the confidence to be themselves and feel beautiful just the way they are.